www.harcourt-internatio

Bringing you products from all Harcourt Health Sciences companies including Baillière Tindall, Churchill Livingstone, Mosby and W.B. Saunders

▶ **Browse** for latest information on new books, journals and electronic products

▶ **Search** for information on over 20 000 published titles with full product information including tables of contents and sample chapters

▶ **Keep up to date** with our extensive publishing programme in your field by registering with eAlert or requesting postal updates

▶ **Secure online ordering** with prompt delivery, as well as full contact details to order by phone, fax or post

▶ **News** of special features and promotions

If you are based in the following countries, please visit the country-specific site to receive full details of product availability and local ordering information

USA: www.harcourthealth.com

Canada: www.harcourtcanada.com

Australia: www.harcourt.com.au

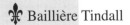 Baillière Tindall   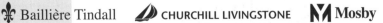 CHURCHILL LIVINGSTONE   Mosby   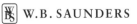 W.B. SAUNDERS

Mind Maps®
in Pathology

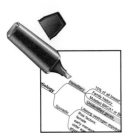

Commissioning Editor: Timothy Horne
Project Development Manager: Siân Jarman
Project Manager: Frances Affleck
Designer: Erik Bigland

Mind Maps® in Pathology

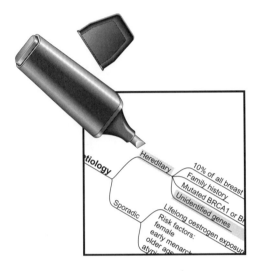

Peter Dervan MD MSc FRCPath
Professor of Pathology
Mater Misericordiae Hospital
University College Dublin
Ireland

Michèle Harrison MD FRCPath
Department of Pathology
Mater Misericordiae Hospital
University College Dublin
Ireland

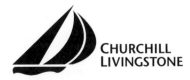
CHURCHILL
LIVINGSTONE

EDINBURGH LONDON NEW YORK PHILADELPHIA ST LOUIS SYDNEY TORONTO 2002

CHURCHILL LIVINGSTONE
An imprint of Harcourt Publishers Limited

© Harcourt Publishers Limited 2002

 is a registered trademark of Harcourt Publishers Limited

First published 2002

ISBN 0-443-07054-7

British Library Cataloguing in Publication Data
A catalogue record for this book is available from the British
Library

Library of Congress Cataloging in Publication Data
A catalog record for this book is available from the Library of
Congress

Mind Map is the Registered Trade Mark of the Buzan
Organisation.

Note
Medical knowledge is constantly changing. As new information
becomes available, changes in treatment, procedures, equipment
and the use of drugs become necessary. The authors and the
publishers have taken care to ensure that the information given
in this text is accurate and up to date. However, readers are
strongly advised to confirm that the information, especially with
regard to drug usage, complies with the latest legislation and
standards of practice.

The
publisher's
policy is to use
**paper manufactured
from sustainable forests**

Printed in China

Preface

Mind Maps in pathology gives an overview of pathology, presented in the form of maps (sometimes called spider maps) with a logical branching format. General pathology (mechanisms of disease) and systemic pathology are covered, with each page being a snapshot of a pathology topic. The branching organisation of the maps highlights the relationships between topics, and places information in a clinical context.

This book should not be used as a stand-alone text. The synopsis format of the book is designed to help the student learn pathology when it is used in conjunction with a standard textbook. In addition, it should facilitate rapid revision for examinations. It should also serve as a useful resource for all healthcare professionals studying or teaching pathology.

Dublin 2002   P. D.
                   M. H.

Acknowledgements

The authors gratefully acknowledge the work of Tony Buzan who devised the concept of Mind Maps, which over many years have proven very helpful to thousands of students in organising their thought processes.

We would also like to acknowledge Mindjet the company whose innovative software allowed us to organise all the Mind Maps in this book. Their website is http://www.mindjet.com/.

Contents

CONTENTS

SYSTEMIC PATHOLOGY

Diseases of infancy and childhood

SYSTEMATIC PATHOLOGY

Cardiovascular system

Respiratory tract

Gastrointestinal tract

Liver, biliary tract and exocrine pancreas

Endocrine system

Kidneys and urinary tract

Male genital tract

Female genital tract

Breast

Blood and bone marrow

Leukaemias and lymphomas

CELLULAR PATHOLOGY

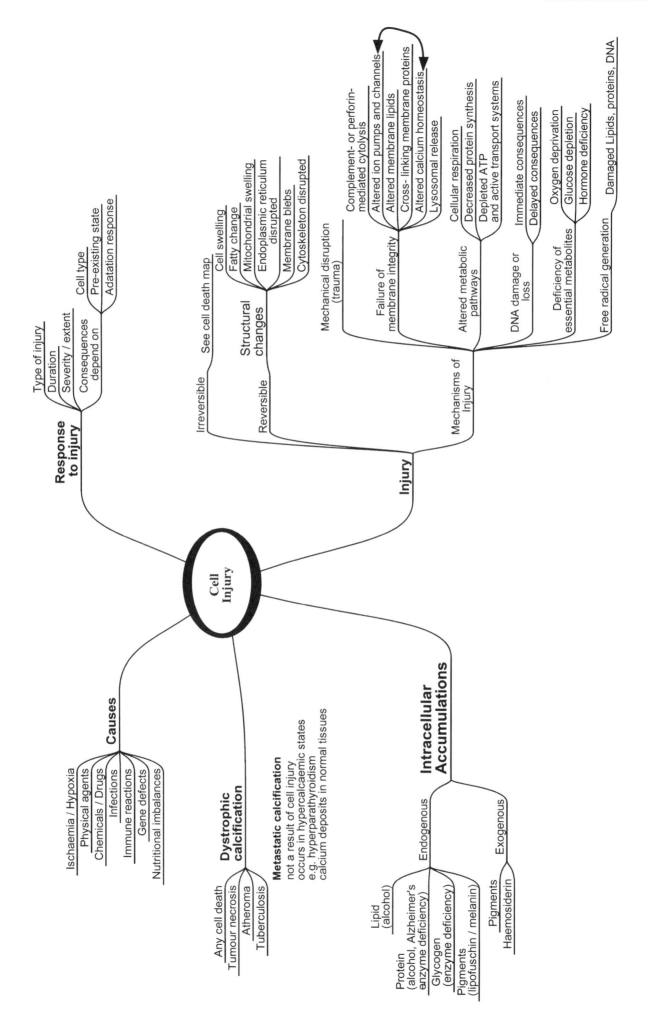

Cell Death

Types of Necrosis

- Involves large group of cells or tissue (part of an organ)
- Necrosis is irreversible
- Coagulative necrosis
- Liquefactive necrosis (colliquative necrosis)
- Caseous necrosis
- Fat necrosis
- Fibrinoid necrosis

Clinical examples of necrosis

- Myocardial infarct, gangrene (coagulative necrosis)
- Brain abscess (liquefactive necrosis)
- Tuberculosis (classic caseous necrosis)
- Acute pancreatitis, breast injury (fat necrosis)
- Malignant hypertension, vasculitis (fibrinoid necrosis blood vessels)

Apoptosis

- Occurs in normal physiological processes (foetus, skin, intestine), or as a result of cell injury
- Apoptosis is irreversible
- Affects single cells (in contrast to necrosis – large tissue mass)
- Pathological processes: (tumours, viral infection, graft v host disease)
- Gene controlled (cell suicide)
  - p53
  - bcl2
- Biochemistry
  - Activated caspases
  - Abnormal protein linking
  - Nucleosome cleaved (200 bp ladder)
  - Cell membrane lipid changes
- Signalling pathways
  - TNF (tumour necrosis factor)
  - Hormones, heat, radiation, hypoxia
  - See cancer genes map for apoptosis regulating genes
- Morphology: cell shrinks, chromatin fragments, cell membrane blebs, phagocytosis, no inflammation

GENERAL PATHOLOGY

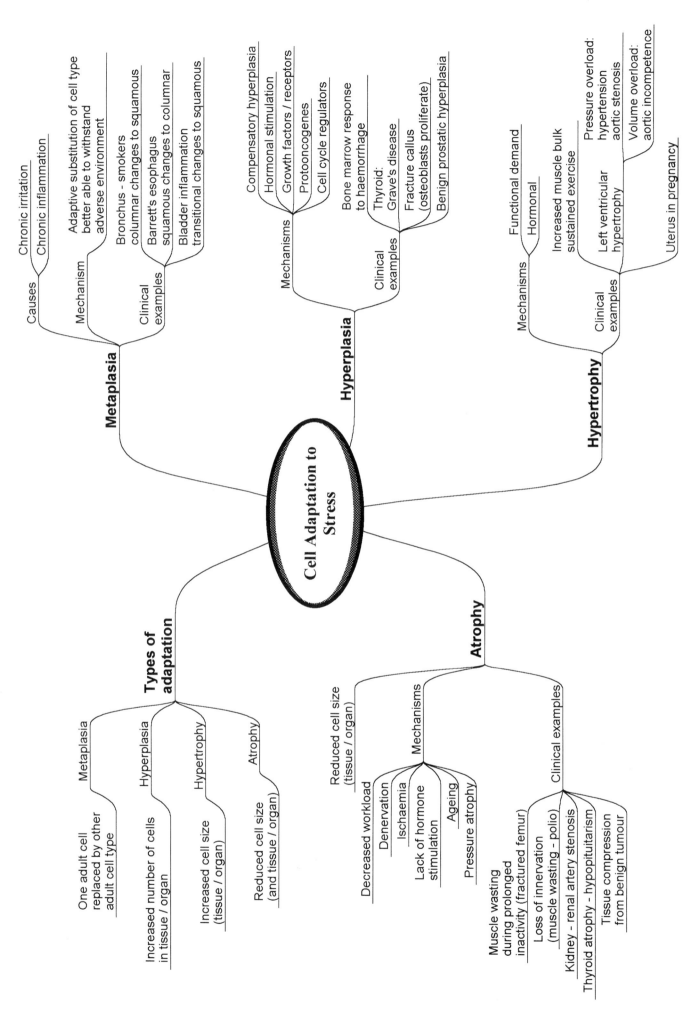

Cell Adaptation to Stress

Metaplasia

Causes
- Chronic irritation
- Chronic inflammation

Mechanism
- Adaptive substitution of cell type better able to withstand adverse environment

Clinical examples
- Bronchus - smokers columnar changes to squamous
- Barrett's esophagus squamous changes to columnar
- Bladder inflammation transitional changes to squamous

Hyperplasia

Mechanisms
- Compensatory hyperplasia
- Hormonal stimulation
- Growth factors / receptors
- Protooncogenes
- Cell cycle regulators

Clinical examples
- Bone marrow response to haemorrhage
- Thyroid: Grave's disease
- Fracture callus (osteoblasts proliferate)
- Benign prostatic hyperplasia

Hypertrophy

Mechanisms
- Functional demand
- Hormonal

Clinical examples
- Increased muscle bulk sustained exercise
- Left ventricular hypertrophy
- Pressure overload: hypertension aortic stenosis
- Volume overload: aortic incompetence
- Uterus in pregnancy

Types of adaptation
- Metaplasia — One adult cell replaced by other adult cell type
- Hyperplasia — Increased number of cells in tissue / organ
- Hypertrophy — Increased cell size (tissue / organ)
- Atrophy — Reduced cell size (and tissue / organ)

Atrophy

Reduced cell size (tissue / organ)

Mechanisms
- Decreased workload
- Denervation
- Ischaemia
- Lack of hormone stimulation
- Ageing
- Pressure atrophy

Clinical examples
- Muscle wasting during prolonged inactivity (fractured femur)
- Loss of innervation (muscle wasting - polio)
- Kidney - renal artery stenosis
- Thyroid atrophy - hypopituitarism
- Tissue compression from benign tumour

GENERAL PATHOLOGY

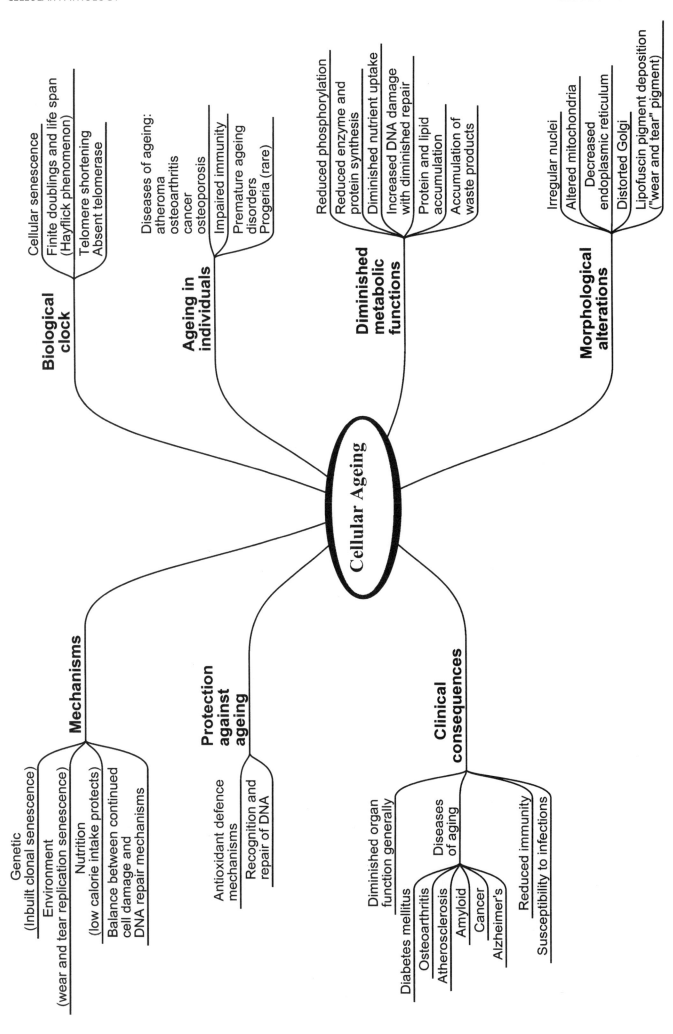

Biological clock

Cellular senescence
Finite doublings and life span (Hayflick phenomenon)
Telomere shortening
Absent telomerase

Ageing in individuals

Diseases of ageing:
atheroma
osteoarthritis
cancer
osteoporosis
Impaired immunity
Premature ageing disorders
Progeria (rare)

Diminished metabolic functions

Reduced phosphorylation
Reduced enzyme and protein synthesis
Diminished nutrient uptake
Increased DNA damage with diminished repair
Protein and lipid accumulation
Accumulation of waste products

Morphological alterations

Irregular nuclei
Altered mitochondria
Decreased endoplasmic reticulum
Distorted Golgi
Lipofuscin pigment deposition ("wear and tear" pigment)

Cellular Ageing

Mechanisms

Genetic (Inbuilt clonal senescence)
Environment (wear and tear replication senescence)
Nutrition (low calorie intake protects)
Balance between continued cell damage and DNA repair mechanisms

Protection against ageing

Antioxidant defence mechanisms
Recognition and repair of DNA

Clinical consequences

Diminished organ function generally
Diseases of aging
Diabetes mellitus
Osteoarthritis
Atherosclerosis
Amyloid
Cancer
Alzheimer's
Reduced immunity
Susceptibility to infections

GENERAL PATHOLOGY

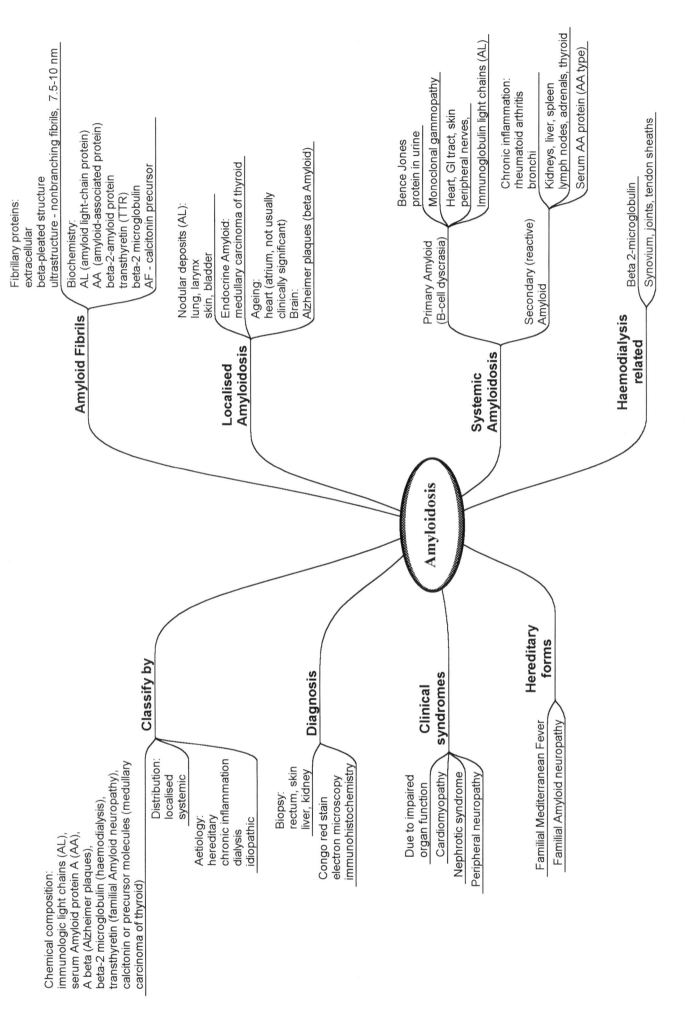

Amyloidosis

Amyloid Fibrils

Fibrillary proteins:
extracellular
beta-pleated structure
ultrastructure - nonbranching fibrils, 7.5-10 nm

Biochemistry:
AL (amyloid light-chain protein)
AA (amyloid-associated protein)
beta-2-amyloid protein
transthyretin (TTR)
beta-2 microglobulin
AF - calcitonin precursor

Localised Amyloidosis

Nodular deposits (AL):
lung, larynx
skin, bladder

Endocrine Amyloid:
medullary carcinoma of thyroid

Ageing:
heart (atrium, not usually
clinically significant)
Brain:
Alzheimer plaques (beta Amyloid)

Systemic Amyloidosis

Bence Jones
protein in urine
Monoclonal gammopathy
Heart, GI tract, skin
peripheral nerves,
Immunoglobulin light chains (AL)

Primary Amyloid
(B-cell dyscrasia)

Chronic inflammation:
rheumatoid arthritis
bronchi
Kidneys, liver, spleen
lymph nodes, adrenals, thyroid
Serum AA protein (AA type)

Secondary (reactive)
Amyloid

Haemodialysis related

Beta 2-microglobulin
Synovium, joints, tendon sheaths

Classify by

Chemical composition:
immunologic light chains (AL),
serum Amyloid protein A (AA),
A beta (Alzheimer plaques),
beta-2 microglobulin (haemodialysis),
transthyretin (familial Amyloid neuropathy),
calcitonin or precursor molecules (medullary
carcinoma of thyroid)

Distribution:
localised
systemic

Aetiology:
hereditary
chronic inflammation
dialysis
idiopathic

Diagnosis

Biopsy:
rectum, skin
liver, kidney

Congo red stain
electron microscopy
immunohistochemistry

Clinical syndromes

Due to impaired
organ function
Cardiomyopathy
Nephrotic syndrome
Peripheral neuropathy

Hereditary forms

Familial Mediterranean Fever
Familial Amyloid neuropathy

ACUTE AND CHRONIC INFLAMMATION

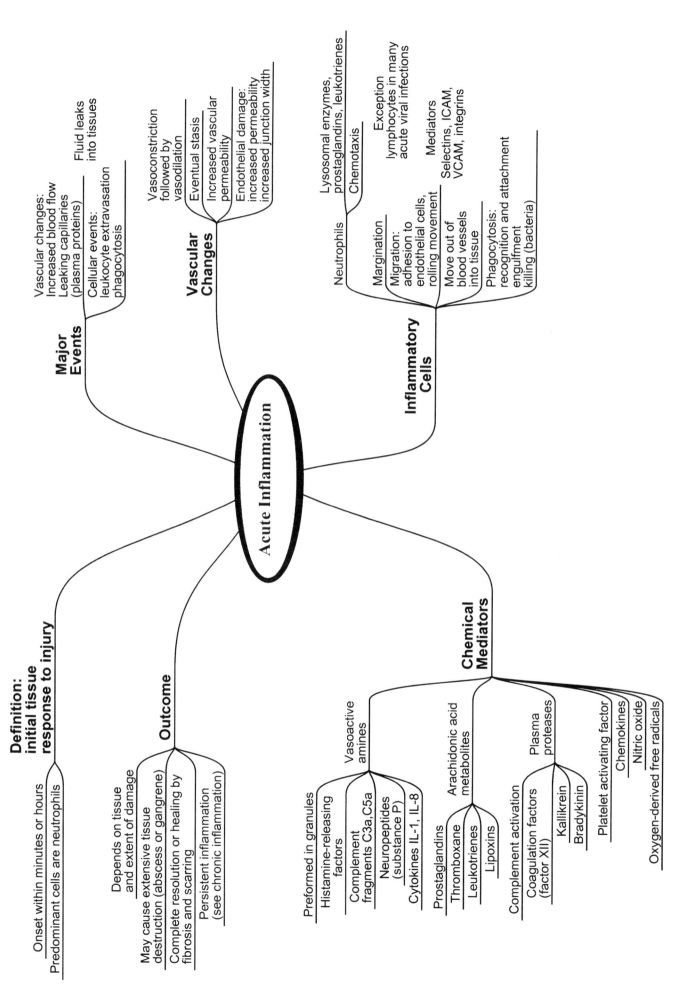

Acute Inflammation

Major Events

Vascular changes:
Increased blood flow
Leaking capillaries
(plasma proteins)

Fluid leaks
into tissues

Cellular events:
leukocyte extravasation
phagocytosis

Vascular Changes

Vasoconstriction
followed by
vasodilation

Eventual stasis

Increased vascular
permeability

Endothelial damage:
increased permeability
increased junction width

Inflammatory Cells

Lysosomal enzymes,
prostaglandins, leukotrienes

Chemotaxis

Neutrophils

Exception
lymphocytes in many
acute viral infections

Mediators
Selectins, ICAM,
VCAM, integrins

Margination

Migration:
adhesion to
endothelial cells,
rolling movement

Move out of
blood vessels
into tissue

Phagocytosis:
recognition and attachment
engulfment
killing (bacteria)

**Definition:
initial tissue
response to injury**

Onset within minutes or hours

Predominant cells are neutrophils

Outcome

Depends on tissue
and extent of damage

May cause extensive tissue
destruction (abscess or gangrene)

Complete resolution or healing by
fibrosis and scarring

Persistent inflammation
(see chronic inflammation)

Chemical Mediators

Vasoactive
amines

Preformed in granules

Histamine-releasing
factors

Complement
fragments C3a, C5a

Neuropeptides
(substance P)

Cytokines IL-1, IL-8

Arachidonic acid
metabolites

Prostaglandins

Thromboxane

Leukotrienes

Lipoxins

Plasma
proteases

Complement activation

Coagulation factors
(factor XII)

Kallikrein

Bradykinin

Platelet activating factor

Chemokines

Nitric oxide

Oxygen-derived free radicals

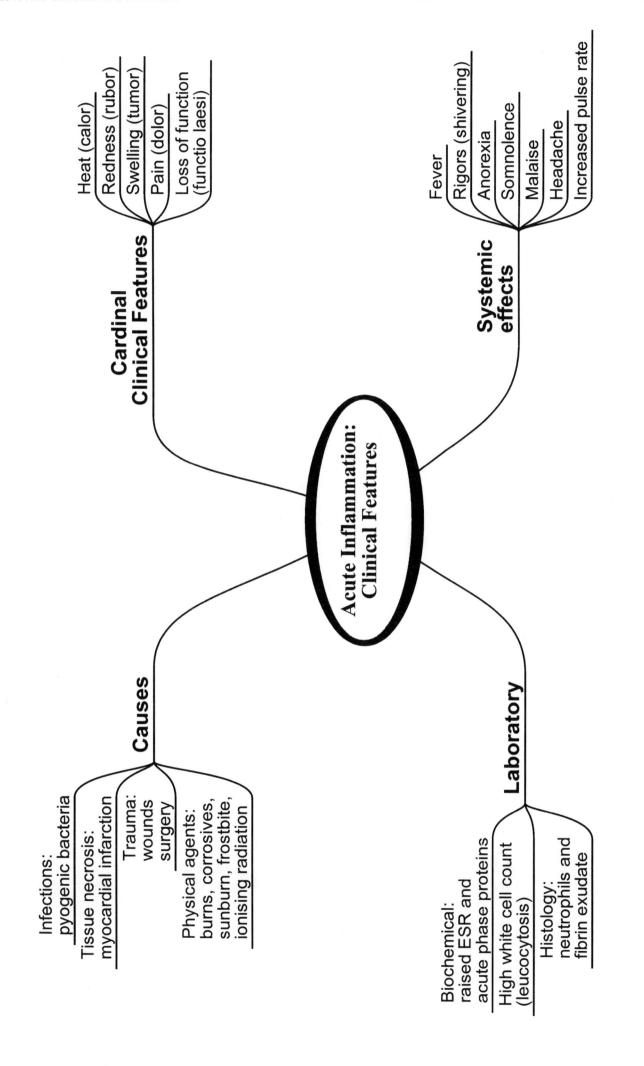

Cardinal Clinical Features
- Heat (calor)
- Redness (rubor)
- Swelling (tumor)
- Pain (dolor)
- Loss of function (functio laesi)

Systemic effects
- Fever
- Rigors (shivering)
- Anorexia
- Somnolence
- Malaise
- Headache
- Increased pulse rate

Acute Inflammation: Clinical Features

Causes
- Infections: pyogenic bacteria
- Tissue necrosis: myocardial infarction
- Trauma: wounds surgery
- Physical agents: burns, corrosives, sunburn, frostbite, ionising radiation

Laboratory
- Biochemical: raised ESR and acute phase proteins
- High white cell count (leucocytosis)
- Histology: neutrophils and fibrin exudate

GENERAL PATHOLOGY

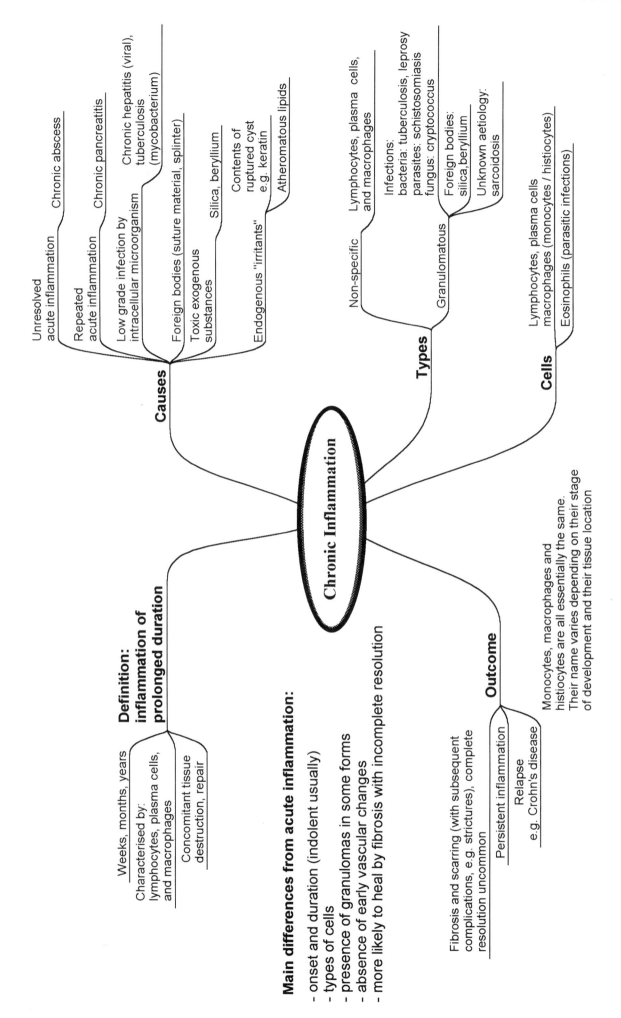

Chronic Inflammation

Causes
- Unresolved acute inflammation → Chronic abscess
- Repeated acute inflammation → Chronic pancreatitis
- Low grade infection by intracellular microorganism → Chronic hepatitis (viral), tuberculosis (mycobacterium)
- Foreign bodies (suture material, splinter)
- Toxic exogenous substances → Silica, beryllium
- Endogenous "irritants" → Contents of ruptured cyst e.g. keratin → Atheromatous lipids

Types
- Non-specific → Lymphocytes, plasma cells, and macrophages
- Granulomatous
  - Infections: bacteria: tuberculosis, leprosy parasites: schistosomiasis fungus: cryptococcus
  - Foreign bodies: silica, beryllium
  - Unknown aetiology: sarcoidosis

Cells
- Lymphocytes, plasma cells
- macrophages (monocytes / histiocytes)
- Eosinophils (parasitic infections)

Monocytes, macrophages and histiocytes are all essentially the same. Their name varies depending on their stage of development and their tissue location

Definition: inflammation of prolonged duration
- Weeks, months, years
- Characterised by: lymphocytes, plasma cells, and macrophages
- Concomitant tissue destruction, repair

Main differences from acute inflammation:

- onset and duration (indolent usually)
- types of cells
- presence of granulomas in some forms
- absence of early vascular changes
- more likely to heal by fibrosis with incomplete resolution

Outcome
- Fibrosis and scarring (with subsequent complications, e.g. strictures), complete resolution uncommon
- Persistent inflammation
- Relapse e.g. Crohn's disease

TISSUE REPAIR

GENERAL PATHOLOGY

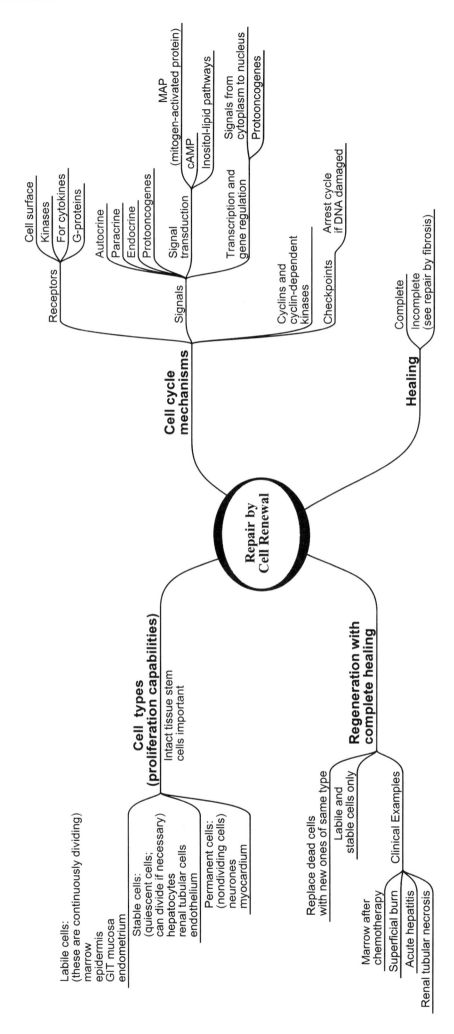

Repair by Cell Renewal

Cell cycle mechanisms

Receptors
- Cell surface
- Kinases
- For cytokines
- G-proteins

Signals
- Autocrine
- Paracrine
- Endocrine
- Protooncogenes

Signal transduction
- cAMP
- MAP (mitogen-activated protein)
- Inositol-lipid pathways

Transcription and gene regulation
- Signals from cytoplasm to nucleus
- Protooncogenes

Cyclins and cyclin-dependent kinases

Checkpoints
- Arrest cycle if DNA damaged

Healing
- Complete
- Incomplete (see repair by fibrosis)

Cell types (proliferation capabilities)

Intact tissue stem cells important

Labile cells: (these are continuously dividing)
- marrow
- epidermis
- GIT mucosa
- endometrium

Stable cells: (quiescent cells; can divide if necessary)
- hepatocytes
- renal tubular cells
- endothelium

Permanent cells: (nondividing cells)
- neurones
- myocardium

Regeneration with complete healing

Replace dead cells with new ones of same type
- Labile and stable cells only

Clinical Examples
- Marrow after chemotherapy
- Superficial burn
- Acute hepatitis
- Renal tubular necrosis

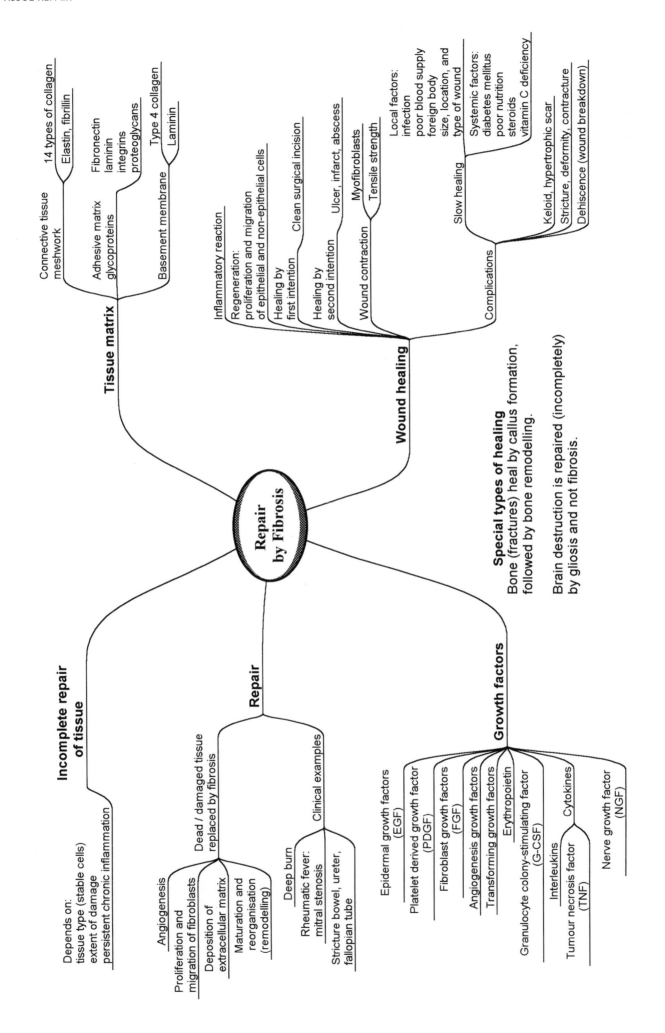

Repair by Fibrosis

Tissue matrix

Connective tissue meshwork
  - 14 types of collagen
  - Elastin, fibrillin

Adhesive matrix glycoproteins
  - Fibronectin
  - laminin
  - integrins
  - proteoglycans

Basement membrane
  - Type 4 collagen
  - Laminin

Wound healing

Inflammatory reaction

Regeneration: proliferation and migration of epithelial and non-epithelial cells

Healing by first intention — Clean surgical incision

Healing by second intention — Ulcer, infarct, abscess

Wound contraction — Myofibroblasts

Tensile strength

Complications
  - Slow healing
    - Local factors: infection, poor blood supply, foreign body, size, location, and type of wound
    - Systemic factors: diabetes mellitus, poor nutrition, steroids, vitamin C deficiency
  - Keloid, hypertrophic scar
  - Stricture, deformity, contracture
  - Dehiscence (wound breakdown)

Special types of healing
Bone (fractures) heal by callus formation, followed by bone remodelling.

Brain destruction is repaired (incompletely) by gliosis and not fibrosis.

Incomplete repair of tissue

Depends on:
  - tissue type (stable cells)
  - extent of damage
  - persistent chronic inflammation

Repair

Angiogenesis

Proliferation and migration of fibroblasts

Deposition of extracellular matrix

Maturation and reorganisation (remodelling)

Dead / damaged tissue replaced by fibrosis

Clinical examples
  - Deep burn
  - Rheumatic fever: mitral stenosis
  - Stricture bowel, ureter, fallopian tube

Growth factors

Epidermal growth factors (EGF)

Platelet derived growth factor (PDGF)

Fibroblast growth factors (FGF)

Angiogenesis growth factors

Transforming growth factors

Erythropoietin

Granulocyte colony-stimulating factor (G-CSF)

Cytokines
  - Interleukins
  - Tumour necrosis factor (TNF)

Nerve growth factor (NGF)

HAEMODYNAMIC DISORDERS, THROMBOSIS AND SHOCK

GENERAL PATHOLOGY

Thrombosis, Embolism and Infarction

Definition of thrombus
Formation of a solid or semi-solid mass from the blood constituents within the vascular system during life

Definition of embolus
Carriage by the bloodstream of material capable of lodging in a blood vessel and thereby obstructing the lumen

Embolism
- 90% derived from thrombi
- Rare forms of emboli - fat, air, atherosclerotic debris, tumour fragments etc.
- Emboli lodge in vessels too small to permit further passage
- Clinical effects depend on the territory supplied by vessel and presence or absence of a collateral circulation

Pulmonary emboli
- Clinical
  - Cause death in 10 - 15% of hospital patients
  - 95% arise from deep venous thrombosis
  - Effects depend on degree of vessel occlusion and state of pulmonary circulation
  - Most are clinically silent
  - Sudden death, right heart failure or cardiovascular collapse occur when > 60% occlusion
  - Medium sized vessel obstruction may result in haemorrhage
  - Multiple emboli may over time -> pulmonary hypertension
  - Symptoms
    - Chest pain
    - Cough
    - Dyspnoea
- Fate of pulmonary emboli
  - Digestion
  - Organisation

Systemic emboli
- Travel through arterial circulation
- Most arise from intracardiac mural thrombi, others from thrombi on atherosclerotic plaques or aortic aneurysms or a valvular vegetation
- Results due to mechanical plugging, major sites - legs, brain, intestine, kidney and spleen

Ischaemia
- Result of impaired vascular perfusion, depriving tissue of vital nutrients
- Effects may be reversible, dependent on the duration of ischaemic episode and the metabolic demands of the tissue

Infarction
- Definition
  - Tissue necrosis resulting from reduction or loss of blood supply
- Most result from thrombosis or embolism
- Pathology
  - Wedge shaped, red or white/pale
  - Initially poorly defined. Become better defined with time due to hyperaemic rim
  - Coagulative necrosis
  - Liquefactive necrosis (brain)
  - Inflammatory response

Thrombosis

Pathogenesis - Virchow's triad
- Endothelial injury
  - Can cause thrombosis by itself
  - Particularly heart and arterial system
  - Caused by haemodynamic stresses eg. hypertension, turbulent blood flow or bacterial toxins
  - Exposure of subendothelial collagen -> adherence of platelets, release of tissue factor etc.
- Alterations in normal blood flow
  - Turbulence and stasis
  - Disrupt normal laminar flow, platelets in contact with endothelium
  - Dilution of activated clotting factors prevented by fresh flowing blood
  - Inflow of clotting factor inhibitors retarded
- Changes in blood constituents
  - Primary hypercoagulability eg. factor V mutations
  - Secondary hypercoagulability eg. oral contraceptives and pregnancy, disseminated cancer, advancing age, smoking and obesity

Pathology
- Anywhere in cardiovascular system
- Variable size and shape, area of attachement to underlying vessel or heart wall
- Platelets, fibrin and blood cells
- Arterial thrombi
  - Site of endothelial injury or turbulence
  - Grow in retrograde direction from site of attachment
  - Lines of Zahn - alternating pale layers of platelets and fibrin and dark layers of red blood cells
  - Mural thrombi - aorta and heart
  - Usually occlusive
- Venous thrombi
  - Sites of stasis
  - Extend in direction of blood flow
  - Resemble coagulated blood
  - Most common in veins of legs
- Vegetations
  - Thrombi may form on heart valves
  - Sterile vegetations - non-bacterial thrombotic endocarditis

Fate of thrombi
- Propagation
- Embolisation
- Dissolution
- Organisation and recanalisation

Clinical effects
- Cause obstruction of arteries and veins
- Possible sources of emboli
- Arterial thrombosis
  - Loss of distal pulses, cold, pale, painful
  - Tissue death and gangrene
- Venous thrombosis
  - Area swollen, reddened and tender

GENERAL PATHOLOGY

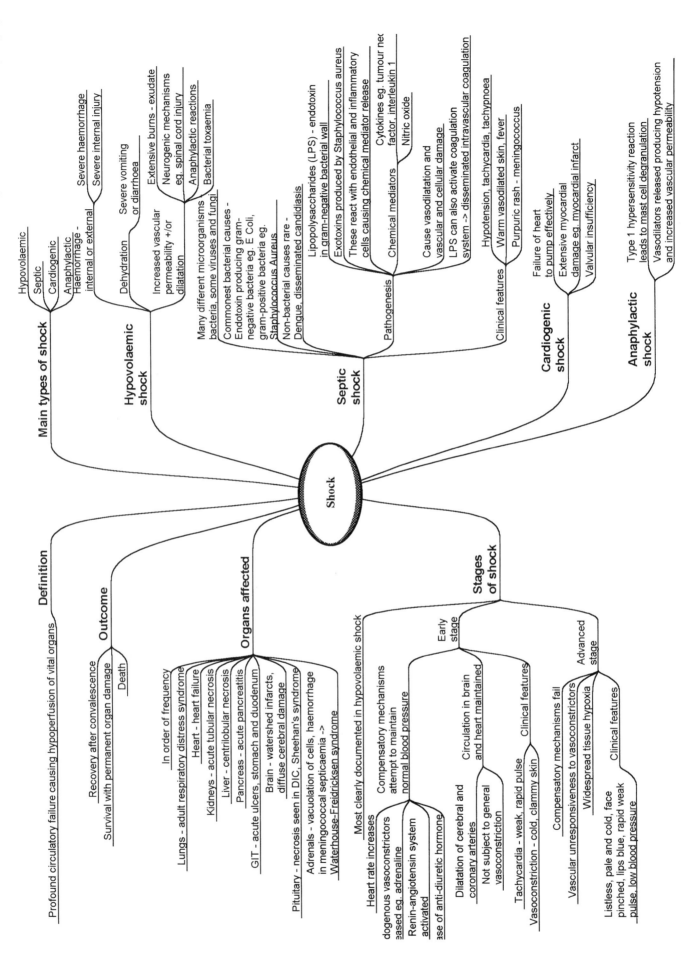

Main types of shock
- Hypovolaemic
- Septic
- Cardiogenic
- Anaphylactic

Hypovolaemic shock
- Haemorrhage - internal or external
  - Severe haemorrhage
  - Severe internal injury
- Dehydration
  - Severe vomiting or diarrhoea
- Increased vascular permeability +/or dilatation
  - Extensive burns - exudate
  - Neurogenic mechanisms eg. spinal cord injury
  - Anaphylactic reactions
  - Bacterial toxaemia

Septic shock
- Many different microorganisms bacteria, some viruses and fungi
  - Commonest bacterial causes - Endotoxin producing gram-negative bacteria eg. E Coli, gram-positive bacteria eg. Staphylococcus Aureus.
  - Non-bacterial causes rare - Dengue, disseminated candidiasis
- Pathogenesis
  - Lipopolysaccharides (LPS) - endotoxin in gram-negative bacterial wall
  - Exotoxins produced by Staphylococcus aureus
  - These react with endothelial and inflammatory cells causing chemical mediator release
  - Chemical mediators
    - Cytokines eg. tumour necrosis factor, interleukin 1
    - Nitric oxide
  - Cause vasodilatation and vascular and cellular damage
  - LPS can also activate coagulation system -> disseminated intravascular coagulation
- Clinical features
  - Hypotension, tachycardia, tachypnoea
  - Warm vasodilated skin, fever
  - Purpuric rash - meningococcus

Cardiogenic shock
- Failure of heart to pump effectively
  - Extensive myocardial damage eg. myocardial infarct
  - Valvular insufficiency

Anaphylactic shock
- Type 1 hypersensitivity reaction leads to mast cell degranulation
- Vasodilators released producing hypotension and increased vascular permeability

Definition
- Profound circulatory failure causing hypoperfusion of vital organs

Outcome
- Recovery after convalescence
- Survival with permanent organ damage
- Death

Organs affected
- In order of frequency
  - Lungs - adult respiratory distress syndrome
  - Heart - heart failure
  - Kidneys - acute tubular necrosis
  - Liver - centrilobular necrosis
  - Pancreas - acute pancreatitis
  - GIT - acute ulcers, stomach and duodenum
  - Brain - watershed infarcts, diffuse cerebral damage
  - Pituitary - necrosis seen in DIC, Sheehan's syndrome
  - Adrenals - vacuolation of cells, haemorrhage in meningococcal septicaemia -> Waterhouse-Freidricksen syndrome

Stages of shock
- Early stage
  - Most clearly documented in hypovolaemic shock
  - Compensatory mechanisms attempt to maintain normal blood pressure
    - Heart rate increases
    - Endogenous vasoconstrictors released eg. adrenaline
    - Renin-angiotensin system activated
    - Release of anti-diuretic hormone
  - Circulation in brain and heart maintained
    - Dilatation of cerebral and coronary arteries
    - Not subject to general vasoconstriction
  - Clinical features
    - Tachycardia - weak, rapid pulse
    - Vasoconstriction - cold, clammy skin
- Advanced stage
  - Compensatory mechanisms fail
    - Vascular unresponsiveness to vasoconstrictors
    - Widespread tissue hypoxia
  - Clinical features
    - Listless, pale and cold, face pinched, lips blue, rapid weak pulse, low blood pressure

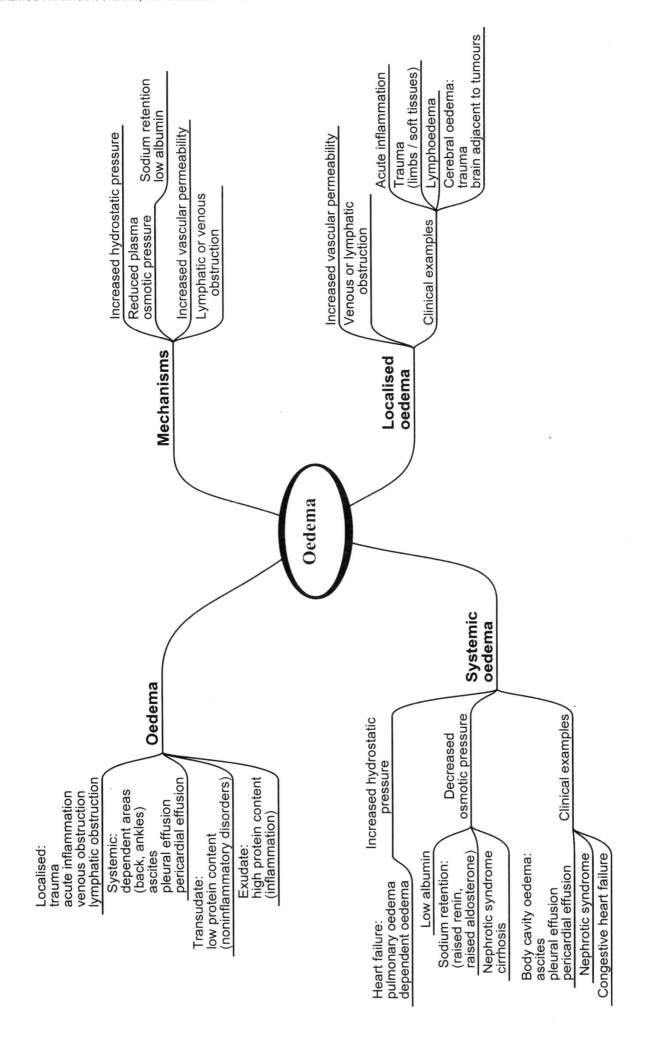

Mechanisms

Increased hydrostatic pressure

Reduced plasma osmotic pressure
- Sodium retention
- low albumin

Increased vascular permeability

Lymphatic or venous obstruction

Localised oedema

Increased vascular permeability

Venous or lymphatic obstruction

Clinical examples
- Acute inflammation
- Trauma (limbs / soft tissues)
- Lymphoedema
- Cerebral oedema: trauma brain adjacent to tumours

Oedema

Oedema

Localised:
- trauma
- acute inflammation
- venous obstruction
- lymphatic obstruction

Systemic:
- dependent areas (back, ankles)
- ascites
- pleural effusion
- pericardial effusion

Transudate:
- low protein content (noninflammatory disorders)

Exudate:
- high protein content (inflammation)

Systemic oedema

Increased hydrostatic pressure

Heart failure:
- pulmonary oedema
- dependent oedema

Decreased osmotic pressure
- Low albumin
- Sodium retention: (raised renin, raised aldosterone)
- Nephrotic syndrome
- cirrhosis

Body cavity oedema:
- ascites
- pleural effusion
- pericardial effusion

Clinical examples
- Nephrotic syndrome
- Congestive heart failure

GENETIC
DISORDERS

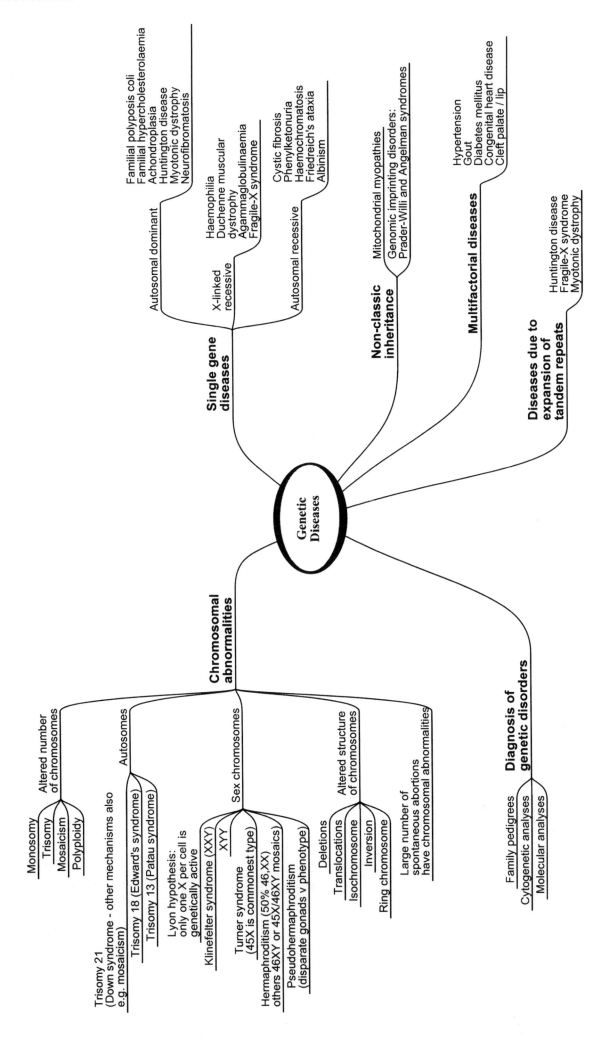

Genetic Diseases

Single gene diseases

Autosomal dominant
- Familial polyposis coli
- Familial hypercholesterolaemia
- Achondroplasia
- Huntington disease
- Myotonic dystrophy
- Neurofibromatosis

X-linked recessive
- Haemophilia
- Duchenne muscular dystrophy
- Agammaglobulinaemia
- Fragile-X syndrome

Autosomal recessive
- Cystic fibrosis
- Phenylketonuria
- Haemochromatosis
- Friedreich's ataxia
- Albinism

Non-classic inheritance
- Mitochondrial myopathies
- Genomic imprinting disorders: Prader-Willi and Angelman syndromes

Multifactorial diseases
- Hypertension
- Gout
- Diabetes mellitus
- Congenital heart disease
- Cleft palate / lip

Diseases due to expansion of tandem repeats
- Huntington disease
- Fragile-X syndrome
- Myotonic dystrophy

Chromosomal abnormalities

Altered number of chromosomes
- Monosomy
- Trisomy
- Mosaicism
- Polyploidy

Autosomes
- Trisomy 21 (Down syndrome - other mechanisms also e.g. mosaicism)
- Trisomy 18 (Edward's syndrome)
- Trisomy 13 (Patau syndrome)

Sex chromosomes
- Lyon hypothesis: only one X per cell is genetically active
- Klinefelter syndrome (XXY)
- XYY
- Turner syndrome (45X is commonest type)
- Hermaphroditism (50% 46,XX) others 46XY or 45X/46XY mosaics)
- Pseudohermaphroditism (disparate gonads v phenotype)

Altered structure of chromosomes
- Deletions
- Translocations
- Isochromosome
- Inversion
- Ring chromosome
- Large number of spontaneous abortions have chromosomal abnormalities

Diagnosis of genetic disorders
- Family pedigrees
- Cytogenetic analyses
- Molecular analyses

GENERAL PATHOLOGY

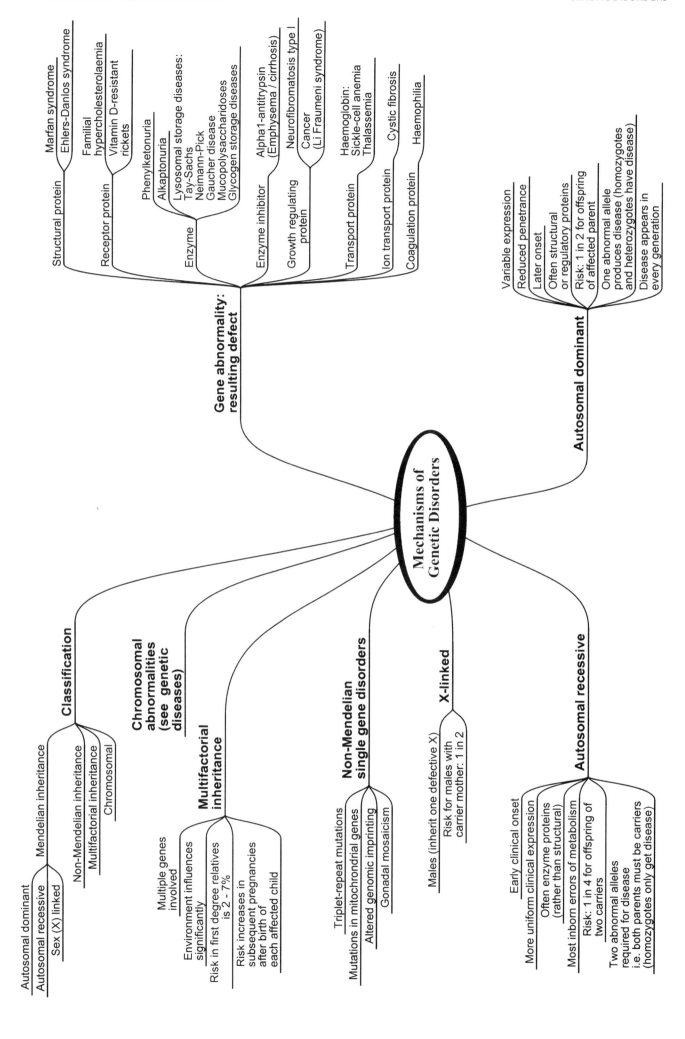

Mechanisms of Genetic Disorders

Gene abnormality: resulting defect

Structural protein
- Marfan syndrome
- Ehlers-Danlos syndrome

Receptor protein
- Familial hypercholesterolaemia
- Vitamin D-resistant rickets

Enzyme
- Phenylketonuria
- Alkaptonuria
- Lysosomal storage diseases:
  - Tay-Sachs
  - Neimann-Pick
  - Gaucher disease
  - Mucopolysaccharidoses
  - Glycogen storage diseases

Enzyme inhibitor
- Alpha1-antitrypsin (Emphysema / cirrhosis)

Growth regulating protein
- Neurofibromatosis type I
- Cancer (Li Fraumeni syndrome)

Transport protein
- Haemoglobin:
  - Sickle-cell anemia
  - Thalassemia

Ion transport protein
- Cystic fibrosis

Coagulation protein
- Haemophilia

Autosomal dominant
- Variable expression
- Reduced penetrance
- Later onset
- Often structural or regulatory proteins
- Risk: 1 in 2 for offspring of affected parent
- One abnormal allele produces disease (homozygotes and heterozygotes have disease)
- Disease appears in every generation

Classification
- Mendelian inheritance
  - Autosomal dominant
  - Autosomal recessive
  - Sex (X) linked
- Non-Mendelian inheritance
- Multifactorial inheritance
- Chromosomal

Chromosomal abnormalities (see genetic diseases)

Multifactorial inheritance
- Multiple genes involved
- Environment influences significantly
- Risk in first degree relatives is 2 - 7%
- Risk increases in subsequent pregnancies after birth of each affected child

Non-Mendelian single gene disorders
- Triplet-repeat mutations
- Mutations in mitochrondrial genes
- Altered genomic imprinting
- Gonadal mosaicism

X-linked
- Males (inherit one defective X)
- Risk for males with carrier mother: 1 in 2

Autosomal recessive
- Early clinical onset
- More uniform clinical expression
- Often enzyme proteins (rather than structural)
- Most inborn errors of metabolism
- Risk: 1 in 4 for offspring of two carriers
- Two abnormal alleles required for disease i.e. both parents must be carriers (homozygotes only get disease)

DISEASES OF IMMUNITY

GENERAL PATHOLOGY

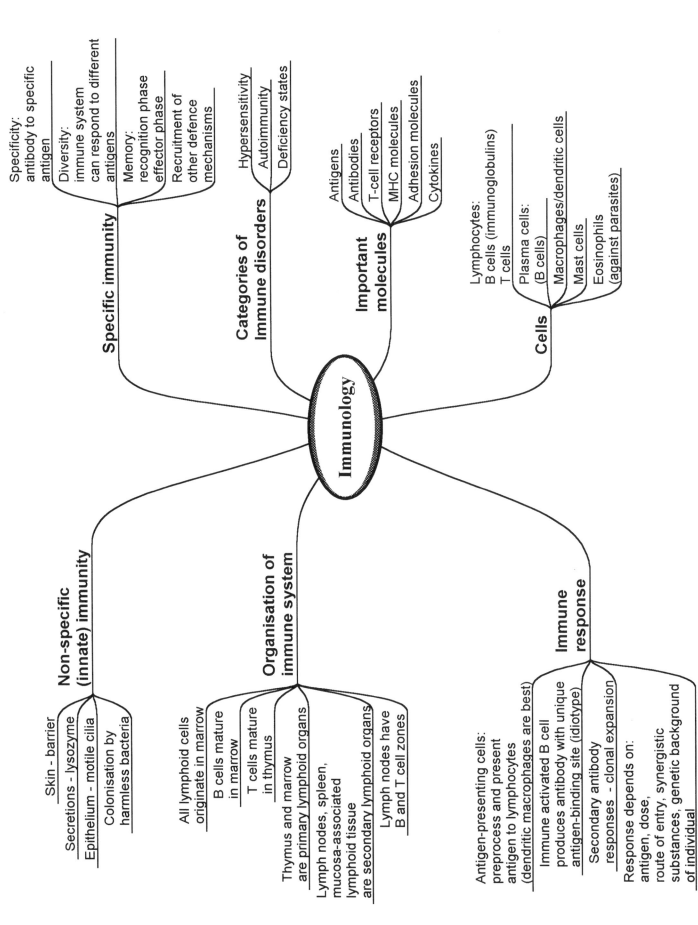

Specific immunity
- Specificity: antibody to specific antigen
- Diversity: immune system can respond to different antigens
- Memory:
  - recognition phase
  - effector phase
- Recruitment of other defence mechanisms

Categories of Immune disorders
- Hypersensitivity
- Autoimmunity
- Deficiency states

Important molecules
- Antigens
- Antibodies
- T-cell receptors
- MHC molecules
- Adhesion molecules
- Cytokines

Cells
- Lymphocytes:
  - B cells (immunoglobulins)
  - T cells
- Plasma cells:
  - (B cells)
- Macrophages/dendritic cells
- Mast cells
- Eosinophils (against parasites)

Immunology

Non-specific (innate) immunity
- Skin - barrier
- Secretions - lysozyme
- Epithelium - motile cilia
- Colonisation by harmless bacteria

Organisation of immune system
- All lymphoid cells originate in marrow
  - B cells mature in marrow
  - T cells mature in thymus
- Thymus and marrow are primary lymphoid organs
- Lymph nodes, spleen, mucosa-associated lymphoid tissue are secondary lymphoid organs
- Lymph nodes have B and T cell zones

Immune response
- Antigen-presenting cells: preprocess and present antigen to lymphocytes (dendritic macrophages are best)
- Immune activated B cell produces antibody with unique antigen-binding site (idiotype)
- Secondary antibody responses - clonal expansion
- Response depends on: antigen, dose, route of entry, synergistic substances, genetic background of individual

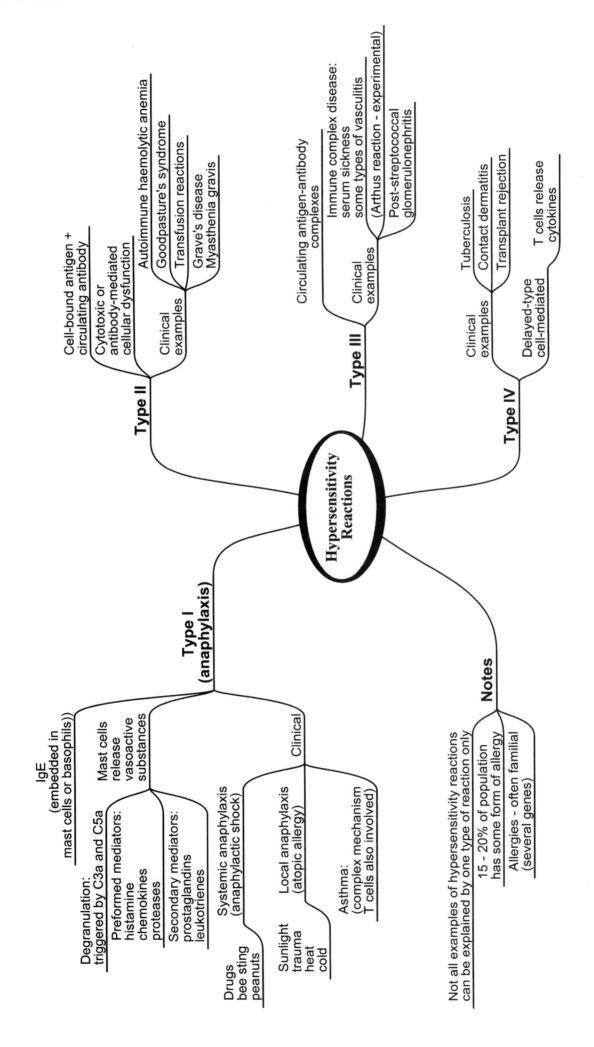

Hypersensitivity Reactions

Type II

Cell-bound antigen + circulating antibody

Cytotoxic or antibody-mediated cellular dysfunction

Clinical examples
- Autoimmune haemolytic anemia
- Goodpasture's syndrome
- Transfusion reactions
- Grave's disease
- Myasthenia gravis

Type III

Circulating antigen-antibody complexes

Clinical examples
- Immune complex disease: serum sickness some types of vasculitis
- (Arthus reaction - experimental)
- Post-streptococcal glomerulonephritis

Type IV

Clinical examples
- Tuberculosis
- Contact dermatitis
- Transplant rejection

Delayed-type cell-mediated
- T cells release cytokines

Type I (anaphylaxis)

IgE (embedded in mast cells or basophils)

Mast cells release vasoactive substances

Degranulation: triggered by C3a and C5a

Preformed mediators:
- histamine
- chemokines
- proteases

Secondary mediators:
- prostaglandins
- leukotrienes

Clinical

Systemic anaphylaxis (anaphylactic shock)
- Drugs
- bee sting
- peanuts

Local anaphylaxis (atopic allergy)
- Sunlight
- trauma
- heat
- cold

Asthma: (complex mechanism T cells also involved)

Notes

Not all examples of hypersensitivity reactions can be explained by one type of reaction only

15 - 20% of population has some form of allergy

Allergies - often familial (several genes)

GENERAL PATHOLOGY

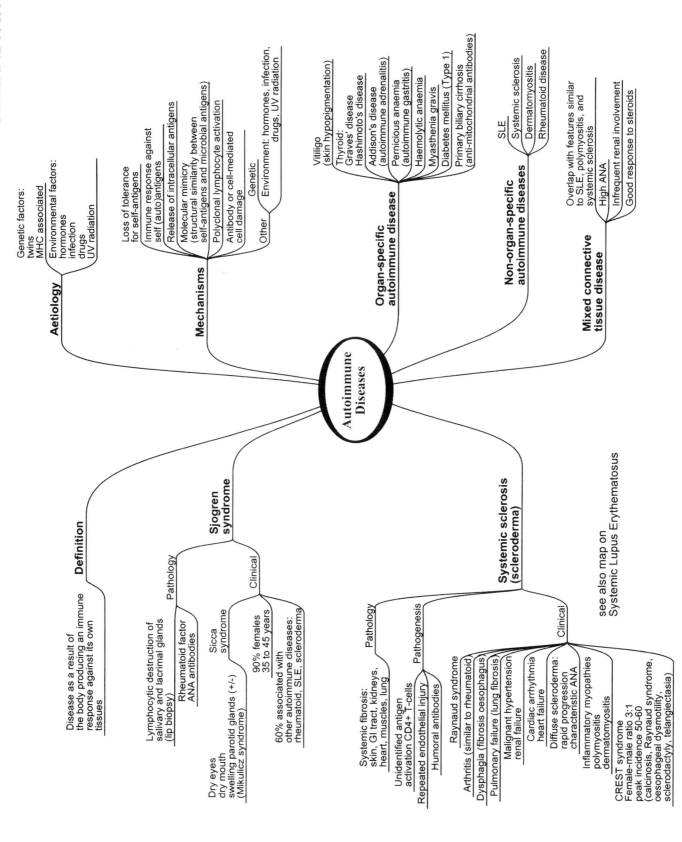

Autoimmune Diseases

Aetiology

Genetic factors:
twins
MHC associated
Environmental factors:
hormones
infection
drugs
UV radiation

Mechanisms

Loss of tolerance for self-antigens
Immune response against self (auto)antigens
Release of intracellular antigens
Molecular mimicry (structural similarity between self-antigens and microbial antigens)
Polyclonal lymphocyte activation
Antibody or cell-mediated cell damage
Genetic
Other
Environment: hormones, infection, drugs, UV radiation

Organ-specific autoimmune disease

Vitiligo (skin hypopigmentation)
Thyroid:
Graves' disease
Hashimoto's disease
Addison's disease (autoimmune adrenalitis)
Pernicious anaemia (autoimmune gastritis)
Haemolytic anaemia
Myasthenia gravis
Diabetes mellitus (Type 1)
Primary biliary cirrhosis (anti-mitochondrial antibodies)

Non-organ-specific autoimmune diseases

SLE
Systemic sclerosis
Dermatomyositis
Rheumatoid disease

Mixed connective tissue disease

Overlap with features similar to SLE, polymyositis, and systemic sclerosis
High ANA
Infrequent renal involvement
Good response to steroids

Definition

Disease as a result of the body producing an immune response against its own tissues

Sjogren syndrome

Pathology
Lymphocytic destruction of salivary and lacrimal glands (lip biopsy)
Rheumatoid factor
ANA antibodies

Clinical
Sicca syndrome
Dry eyes
dry mouth
swelling parotid glands (+/-) (Mikulicz syndrome)
90% females
35 to 45 years
60% associated with other autoimmune diseases: rheumatoid, SLE, scleroderma

Systemic sclerosis (scleroderma)

Pathology
Systemic fibrosis: skin, GI tract, kidneys, heart, muscles, lung

Pathogenesis
Unidentified antigen activation CD4+ T-cells
Repeated endothelial injury
Humoral antibodies

Clinical
Raynaud syndrome
Arthritis (similar to rheumatoid)
Dysphagia (fibrosis oesophagus)
Pulmonary failure (lung fibrosis)
Malignant hypertension renal failure
Cardiac arrhythmia heart failure
Diffuse scleroderma: rapid progression characteristic ANA
Inflammatory myopathies polymyositis dermatomyositis
CREST syndrome
Female-male ratio 3:1
peak incidence 50-60
(calcinosis, Raynaud syndrome, oesophageal dysmotility, sclerodactyly, telangiectasia)

see also map on Systemic Lupus Erythematosus

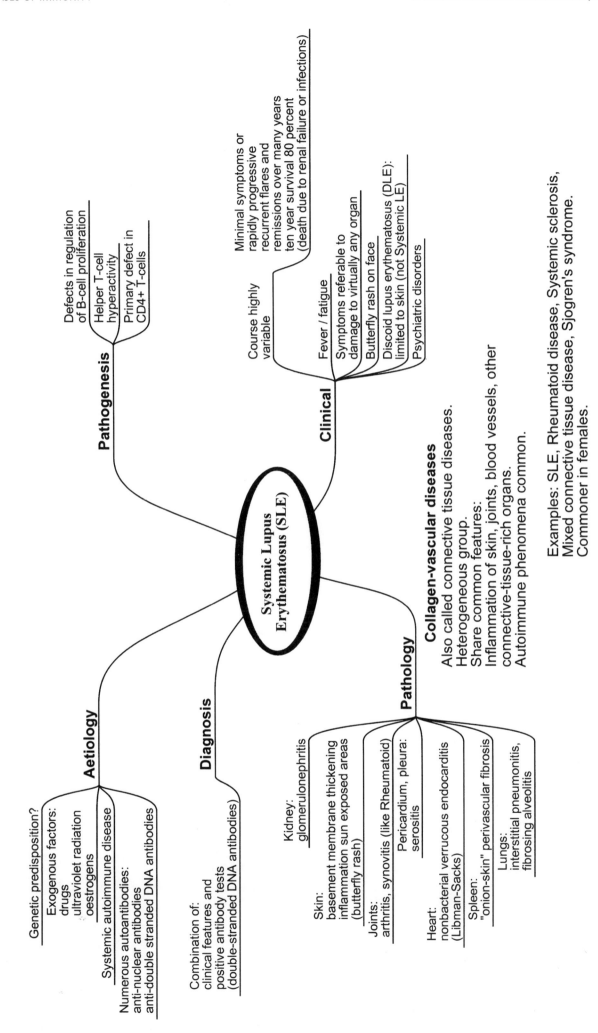

Systemic Lupus Erythematosus (SLE)

Pathogenesis

Defects in regulation of B-cell proliferation
- Helper T-cell hyperactivity
- Primary defect in CD4+ T-cells

Clinical

Course highly variable
- Minimal symptoms or rapidly progressive recurrent flares and remissions over many years ten year survival 80 percent (death due to renal failure or infections)

- Fever / fatigue
- Symptoms referable to damage to virtually any organ
- Butterfly rash on face
- Discoid lupus erythematosus (DLE): limited to skin (not Systemic LE)
- Psychiatric disorders

Aetiology

Genetic predisposition?
- Exogenous factors:
  drugs
  ultraviolet radiation
  oestrogens
- Systemic autoimmune disease

Numerous autoantibodies:
anti-nuclear antibodies
anti-double stranded DNA antibodies

Diagnosis

Combination of:
clinical features and
positive antibody tests
(double-stranded DNA antibodies)

Pathology

Collagen-vascular diseases

Also called connective tissue diseases.
Heterogeneous group.
Share common features:
Inflammation of skin, joints, blood vessels, other connective-tissue-rich organs.
Autoimmune phenomena common.

Examples: SLE, Rheumatoid disease, Systemic sclerosis, Mixed connective tissue disease, Sjogren's syndrome.
Commoner in females.

Kidney:
glomerulonephritis

Skin:
basement membrane thickening inflammation sun exposed areas (butterfly rash)

Joints:
arthritis, synovitis (like Rheumatoid)

Heart:
nonbacterial verrucous endocarditis (Libman-Sacks)

Pericardium, pleura: serositis

Spleen:
"onion-skin" perivascular fibrosis

Lungs:
interstitial pneumonitis, fibrosing alveolitis

GENERAL PATHOLOGY

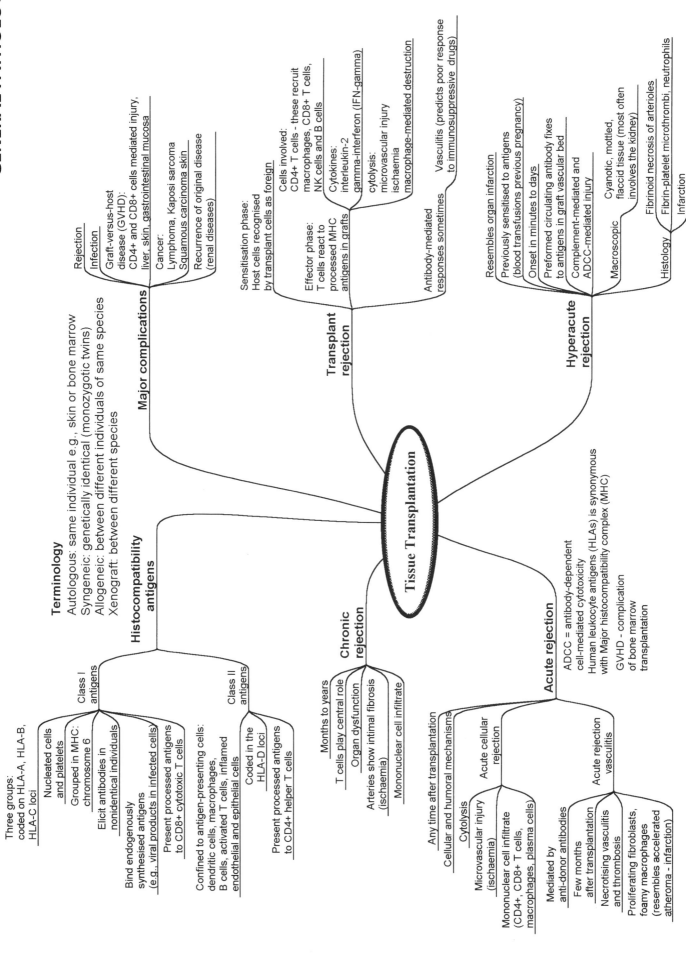

Tissue Transplantation

Major complications

Rejection

Infection

Graft-versus-host disease (GVHD): CD4+ and CD8+ cells mediated injury, liver, skin, gastrointestinal mucosa

Cancer: Lymphoma, Kaposi sarcoma Squamous carcinoma skin

Recurrence of original disease (renal diseases)

Transplant rejection

Sensitisation phase: Host cells recognised by transplant cells as foreign

Effector phase: T cells react to processed MHC antigens in grafts

Cells involved: CD4+ T cells - these recruit macrophages, CD8+ T cells, NK cells and B cells

Cytokines: interleukin-2 gamma-interferon (IFN-gamma)

cytolysis: microvascular injury ischaemia macrophage-mediated destruction

Antibody-mediated responses sometimes

Vasculitis (predicts poor response to immunosuppressive drugs)

Hyperacute rejection

Resembles organ infarction

Previously sensitised to antigens (blood transfusions previous pregnancy)

Onset in minutes to days

Preformed circulating antibody fixes to antigens in graft vascular bed

Complement-mediated and ADCC-mediated injury

Macroscopic: Cyanotic, mottled, flaccid tissue (most often involves the kidney)

Histology: Fibrinoid necrosis of arterioles

Fibrin-platelet microthrombi; neutrophils

Infarction

Terminology

Autologous: same individual e.g., skin or bone marrow
Syngeneic: genetically identical (monozygotic twins)
Allogeneic: between different individuals of same species
Xenograft: between different species

Histocompatibility antigens

Three groups: coded on HLA-A, HLA-B, HLA-C loci

Nucleated cells and platelets

Grouped in MHC: chromosome 6

Elicit antibodies in nonidentical individuals

Class I antigens

Bind endogenously synthesised antigens (e.g., viral products in infected cells)

Present processed antigens to CD8+ cytotoxic T cells

Confined to antigen-presenting cells: dendritic cells, macrophages, B cells, activated T cells, inflamed endothelial and epithelial cells

Class II antigens

Coded in the HLA-D loci

Present processed antigens to CD4+ helper T cells

Chronic rejection

Months to years

T cells play central role

Organ dysfunction

Arteries show intimal fibrosis (ischaemia)

Mononuclear cell infiltrate

Acute rejection

ADCC = antibody-dependent cell-mediated cytotoxicity

Human leukocyte antigens (HLAs) is synonymous with Major histocompatibility complex (MHC)

GVHD - complication of bone marrow transplantation

Any time after transplantation

Cellular and humoral mechanisms

Acute cellular rejection

Cytolysis

Microvascular injury (ischaemia)

Mononuclear cell infiltrate (CD4+, CD8+ T cells, macrophages, plasma cells)

Acute rejection vasculitis

Mediated by anti-donor antibodies

Few months after transplantation

Necrotising vasculitis and thrombosis

Proliferating fibroblasts, foamy macrophages (resembles accelerated atheroma - infarction)

GENERAL PATHOLOGY

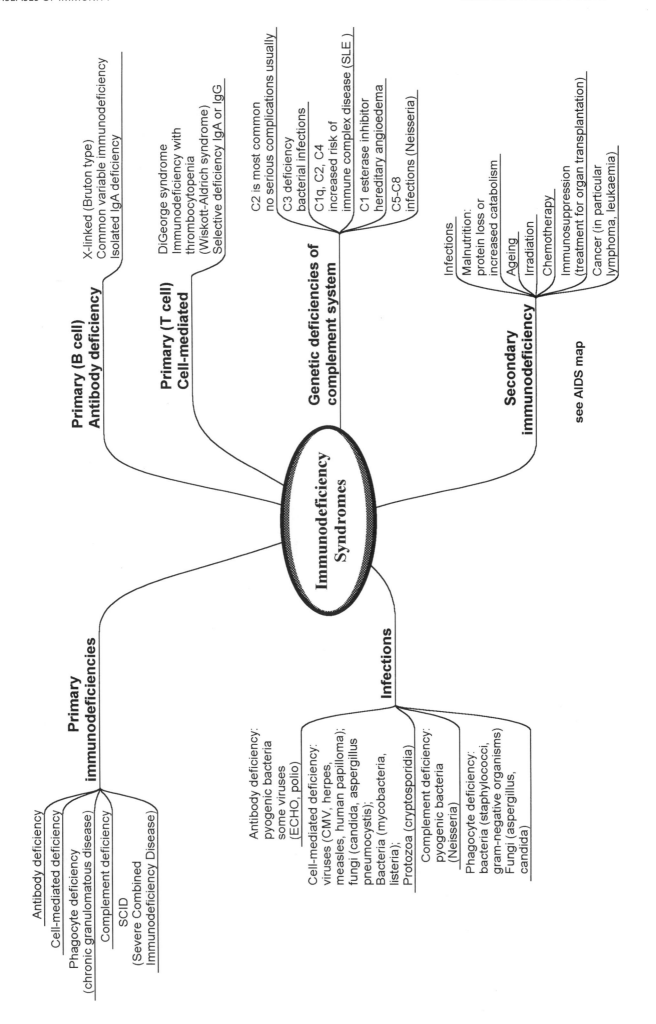

Primary (B cell) Antibody deficiency
- X-linked (Bruton type)
- Common variable immunodeficiency
- Isolated IgA deficiency

Primary (T cell) Cell-mediated
- DiGeorge syndrome
- Immunodeficiency with thrombocytopenia (Wiskott-Aldrich syndrome)
- Selective deficiency IgA or IgG

Genetic deficiencies of complement system
- C2 is most common no serious complications usually
- C3 deficiency bacterial infections
- C1q, C2, C4 increased risk of immune complex disease (SLE)
- C1 esterase inhibitor hereditary angioedema
- C5-C8 infections (Neisseria)

Secondary immunodeficiency
- Infections
- Malnutrition: protein loss or increased catabolism
- Ageing
- Irradiation
- Chemotherapy
- Immunosuppression (treatment for organ transplantation)
- Cancer (in particular lymphoma, leukaemia)

see AIDS map

Immunodeficiency Syndromes

Primary immunodeficiencies
- Antibody deficiency
- Cell-mediated deficiency
- Phagocyte deficiency (chronic granulomatous disease)
- Complement deficiency
- SCID (Severe Combined Immunodeficiency Disease)

Infections
- Antibody deficiency: pyogenic bacteria some viruses (ECHO, polio)
- Cell-mediated deficiency: viruses (CMV, herpes, measles, human papilloma); fungi (candida, aspergillus pneumocystis); Bacteria (mycobacteria, listeria); Protozoa (cryptosporidia)
- Complement deficiency: pyogenic bacteria (Neisseria)
- Phagocyte deficiency: bacteria (staphylococci, gram-negative organisms) Fungi (aspergillus, candida)

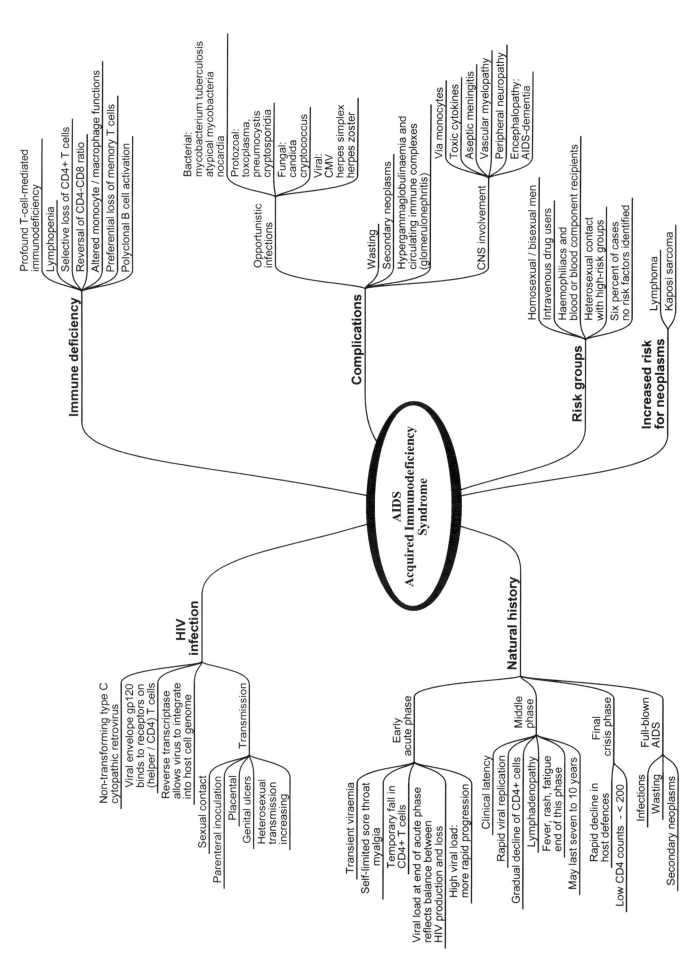

Immune deficiency

- Profound T-cell-mediated immunodeficiency
- Lymphopenia
- Selective loss of CD4+ T cells
- Reversal of CD4-CD8 ratio
- Altered monocyte / macrophage functions
- Preferential loss of memory T cells
- Polyclonal B cell activation

Complications

- Opportunistic infections
  - Bacterial: mycobacterium tuberculosis, atypical mycobacteria, nocardia
  - Protozoal: toxoplasma, pneumocystis, cryptosporidia
  - Fungal: candida, cryptococcus
  - Viral: CMV, herpes simplex, herpes zoster
- Wasting
- Secondary neoplasms
- Hypergammaglobulinaemia and circulating immune complexes (glomerulonephritis)
- CNS involvement
  - Via monocytes
  - Toxic cytokines
  - Aseptic meningitis
  - Vascular myelopathy
  - Peripheral neuropathy
  - Encephalopathy: AIDS-dementia

Risk groups

- Homosexual / bisexual men
- Intravenous drug users
- Haemophiliacs and blood or blood component recipients
- Heterosexual contact with high-risk groups
- Six percent of cases no risk factors identified

Increased risk for neoplasms

- Lymphoma
- Kaposi sarcoma

AIDS Acquired Immunodeficiency Syndrome

HIV infection

- Non-transforming type C cytopathic retrovirus
- Viral envelope gp120 binds to receptors on (helper / CD4) T cells
- Reverse transcriptase allows virus to integrate into host cell genome
- Transmission
  - Sexual contact
  - Parenteral inoculation
  - Placental
  - Genital ulcers
  - Heterosexual transmission increasing

Natural history

- Early acute phase
  - Transient viraemia
  - Self-limited sore throat myalgia
  - Temporary fall in CD4+ T cells
  - Viral load at end of acute phase reflects balance between HIV production and loss
  - High viral load: more rapid progression
- Middle phase
  - Clinical latency
  - Rapid viral replication
  - Gradual decline of CD4+ cells
  - Lymphadenopathy
  - Fever, rash, fatigue end of this phase
  - May last seven to 10 years
- Final crisis phase
  - Rapid decline in host defences
  - Low CD4 counts - < 200
- Full-blown AIDS
  - Infections
  - Wasting
  - Secondary neoplasms

GENERAL PATHOLOGY

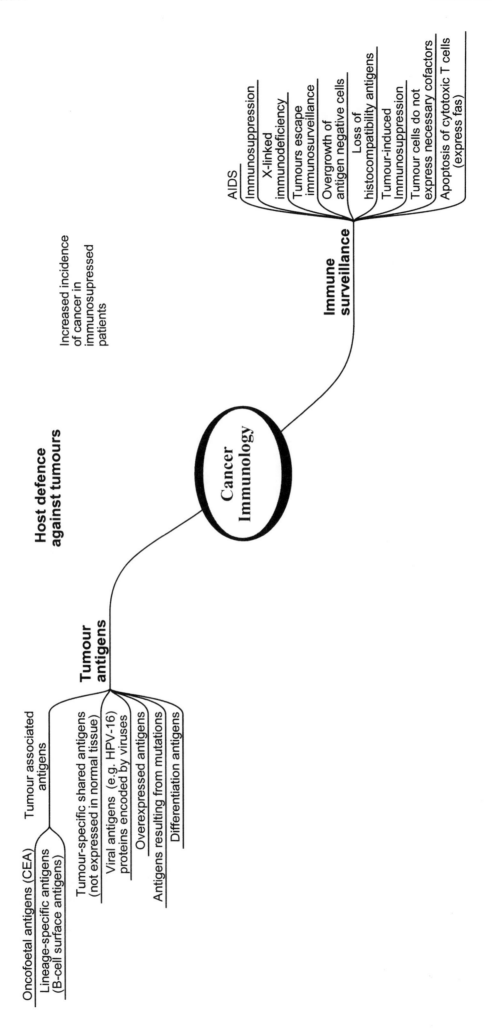

Host defence against tumours

Increased incidence of cancer in immunosupressed patients

Tumour antigens

Oncofoetal antigens (CEA)

Tumour associated antigens

Lineage-specific antigens (B-cell surface antigens)

Tumour-specific shared antigens (not expressed in normal tissue)

Viral antigens (e.g. HPV-16) proteins encoded by viruses

Overexpressed antigens

Antigens resulting from mutations

Differentiation antigens

Cancer Immunology

Immune surveillance

AIDS

Immunosuppression

X-linked immunodeficiency

Tumours escape immunosurveillance

Overgrowth of antigen negative cells

Loss of histocompatibility antigens

Tumour-induced Immunosuppression

Tumour cells do not express necessary cofactors

Apoptosis of cytotoxic T cells (express fas)

NEOPLASIA

GENERAL PATHOLOGY

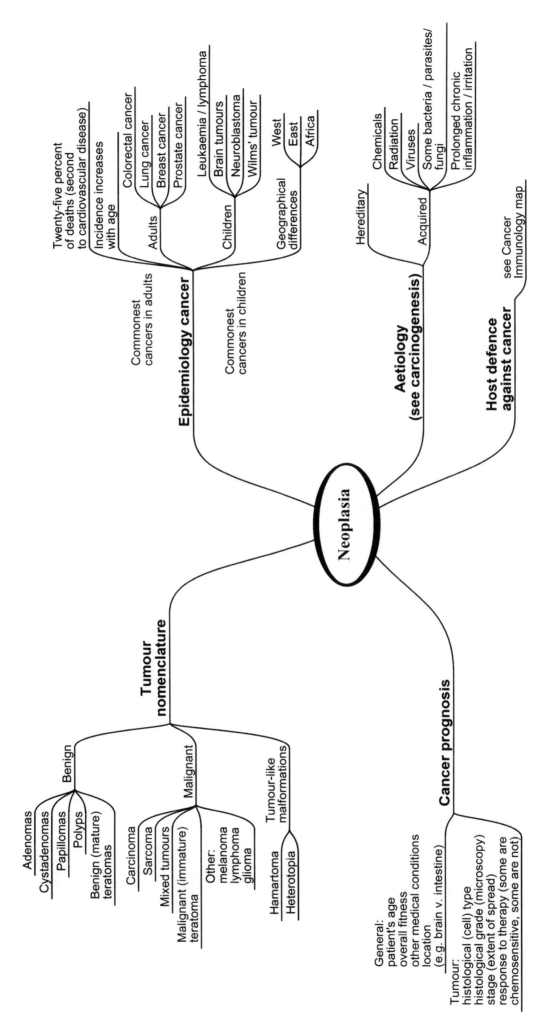

Neoplasia

Epidemiology cancer

Commonest cancers in adults
- Twenty-five percent of deaths (second to cardiovascular disease)
- Incidence increases with age
- Adults
  - Colorectal cancer
  - Lung cancer
  - Breast cancer
  - Prostate cancer

Commonest cancers in children
- Children
  - Leukaemia / lymphoma
  - Brain tumours
  - Neuroblastoma
  - Wilms' tumour
- Geographical differences
  - West
  - East
  - Africa

Aetiology (see carcinogenesis)
- Hereditary
- Acquired
  - Chemicals
  - Radiation
  - Viruses
  - Some bacteria / parasites / fungi
  - Prolonged chronic inflammation / irritation

Host defence against cancer
- see Cancer Immunology map

Tumour nomenclature
- Benign
  - Adenomas
  - Cystadenomas
  - Papillomas
  - Polyps
  - Benign (mature) teratomas
- Malignant
  - Carcinoma
  - Sarcoma
  - Mixed tumours
  - Malignant (immature) teratoma
  - Other: melanoma lymphoma glioma
- Tumour-like malformations
  - Hamartoma
  - Heterotopia

Cancer prognosis
- General: patient's age overall fitness other medical conditions location (e.g. brain v. intestine)
- Tumour: histological (cell) type histological grade (microscopy) stage (extent of spread) response to therapy (some are chemosensitive, some are not)

GENERAL PATHOLOGY

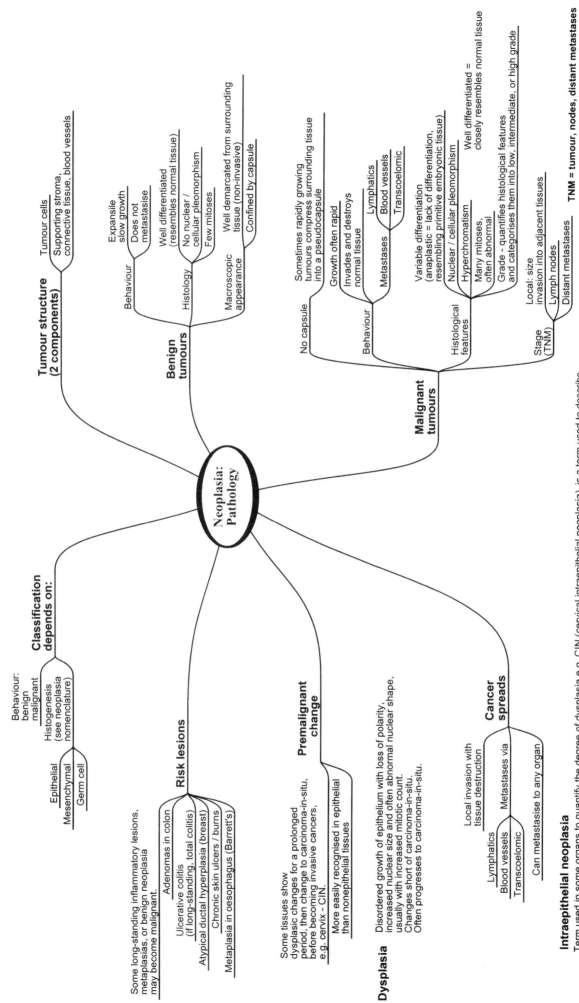

Tumour structure (2 components)
- Tumour cells
- Supporting stroma, connective tissue, blood vessels

Benign tumours
- Behaviour
  - Expansile slow growth
  - Does not metastasise
- Histology
  - Well differentiated (resembles normal tissue)
  - No nuclear / cellular pleomorphism
  - Few mitoses
- Macroscopic appearance
  - Well demarcated from surrounding tissue (non-invasive)
  - Confined by capsule

Malignant tumours
- No capsule
  - Sometimes rapidly growing tumours compress surrounding tissue into a pseudocapsule
- Behaviour
  - Growth often rapid
  - Invades and destroys normal tissue
  - Metastases
    - Lymphatics
    - Blood vessels
    - Transcoelomic
- Histological features
  - Variable differentiation (anaplastic = lack of differentiation, resembling primitive embryonic tissue)
  - Nuclear / cellular pleomorphism
  - Hyperchromatism
  - Many mitoses, often abnormal
  - Grade - quantifies histological features and categorises them into low, intermediate, or high grade
  - Well differentiated = closely resembles normal tissue
- Stage (TNM)
  - Local: size invasion into adjacent tissues
  - Lymph nodes
  - Distant metastases

TNM = tumour, nodes, distant metastases

Classification depends on:
- Behaviour: benign malignant
- Histogenesis (see neoplasia nomenclature)
  - Epithelial
  - Mesenchymal
  - Germ cell

Risk lesions

Some long-standing inflammatory lesions, metaplasias, or benign neoplasia may become malignant.
- Adenomas in colon
- Ulcerative colitis (if long-standing, total colitis)
- Atypical ductal hyperplasia (breast)
- Chronic skin ulcers / burns
- Metaplasia in oesophagus (Barrett's)

Premalignant change

Some tissues show dysplasic changes for a prolonged period, then change to carcinoma-in-situ, before becoming invasive cancers, e.g. cervix - CIN.

More easily recognised in epithelial than nonepithelial tissues

Dysplasia
Disordered growth of epithelium with loss of polarity, increased nuclear size and often abnormal nuclear shape, usually with increased mitotic count.
Changes short of carcinoma-in-situ.
Often progresses to carcinoma-in-situ.

Cancer spreads
- Local invasion with tissue destruction
- Metastases via
  - Lymphatics
  - Blood vessels
  - Transcoelomic
- Can metastasise to any organ

Intraepithelial neoplasia
Term used in some organs to quantify the degree of dysplasia e.g. CIN (cervical intraepithelial neoplasia), is a term used to describe dysplasia or carcinoma-in-situ in the cervix. CIN I refers to low grade dysplasia; CIN III refers to high grade dysplasia and carcinoma-in-situ (it does not distinguish between them - in clinical practice they have the same significance)

Neoplasia: Pathology

GENERAL PATHOLOGY

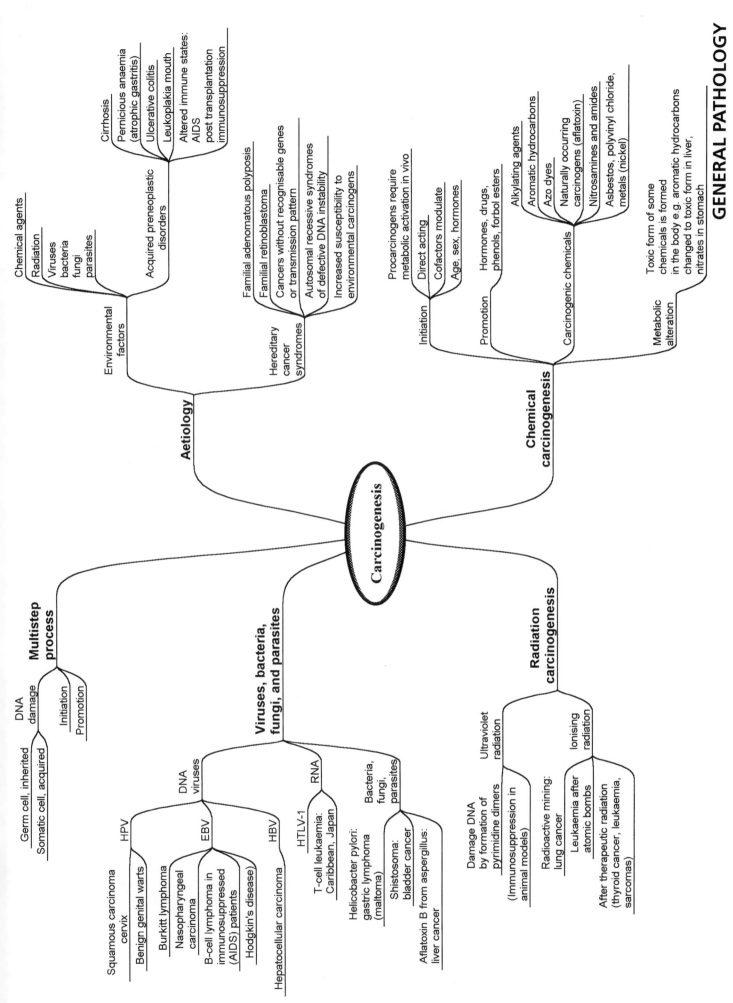

Carcinogenesis

Aetiology

Environmental factors
- Chemical agents
- Radiation
- Viruses bacteria fungi parasites

Acquired preneoplastic disorders
- Cirrhosis
- Pernicious anaemia (atrophic gastritis)
- Ulcerative colitis
- Leukoplakia mouth
- Altered immune states: AIDS post transplantation immunosuppression

Hereditary cancer syndromes
- Familial adenomatous polyposis
- Familial retinoblastoma
- Cancers without recognisable genes or transmission pattern
- Autosomal recessive syndromes of defective DNA instability
- Increased susceptibility to environmental carcinogens

Chemical carcinogenesis

Initiation
- Procarcinogens require metabolic activation in vivo
- Direct acting
- Cofactors modulate
- Age, sex, hormones

Promotion
- Hormones, drugs, phenols, forbol esters

Carcinogenic chemicals
- Alkylating agents
- Aromatic hydrocarbons
- Azo dyes
- Naturally occurring carcinogens (aflatoxin)
- Nitrosamines and amides
- Asbestos, polyvinyl chloride, metals (nickel)

Metabolic alteration
- Toxic form of some chemicals is formed in the body e.g. aromatic hydrocarbons changed to toxic form in liver, nitrates in stomach

Multistep process

DNA damage
- Germ cell, inherited
- Somatic cell, acquired

- Initiation
- Promotion

Viruses, bacteria, fungi, and parasites

DNA viruses
- HPV
  - Squamous carcinoma cervix
  - Benign genital warts
- EBV
  - Burkitt lymphoma
  - Nasopharyngeal carcinoma
  - B-cell lymphoma in immunosuppressed (AIDS) patients
  - Hodgkin's disease)
- HBV
  - Hepatocellular carcinoma

RNA
- HTLV-1
  - T-cell leukaemia: Caribbean, Japan

Bacteria, fungi, parasites
- Helicobacter pylori: gastric lymphoma (maltoma)
- Shistosoma: bladder cancer
- Aflatoxin B from aspergillus: liver cancer

Radiation carcinogenesis

Ultraviolet radiation
- Damage DNA by formation of pyrimidine dimers
- (Immunosuppression in animal models)

Ionising radiation
- Radioactive mining: lung cancer
- Leukaemia after atomic bombs
- After therapeutic radiation (thyroid cancer, leukaemia, sarcomas)

GENERAL PATHOLOGY

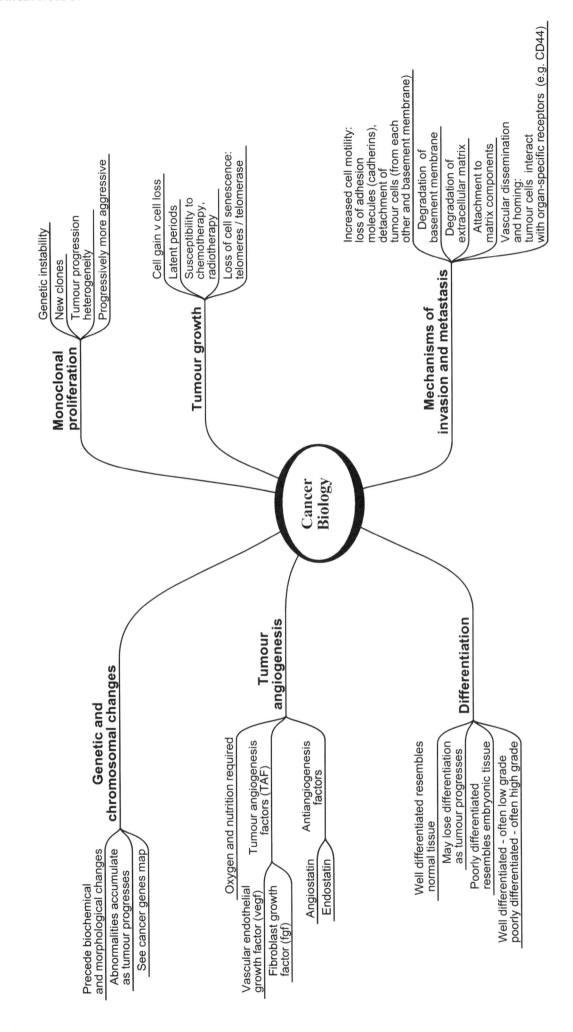

Cancer Biology

Monoclonal proliferation
- Genetic instability
- New clones
- Tumour progression heterogeneity
- Progressively more aggressive

Tumour growth
- Cell gain v cell loss
- Latent periods
- Susceptibility to chemotherapy, radiotherapy
- Loss of cell senescence: telomeres / telomerase

Mechanisms of invasion and metastasis
- Increased cell motility: loss of adhesion molecules (cadherins), detachment of tumour cells (from each other and basement membrane)
- Degradation of basement membrane
- Degradation of extracellular matrix
- Attachment to matrix components
- Vascular dissemination and homing: tumour cells interact with organ-specific receptors (e.g. CD44)

Genetic and chromosomal changes
- Precede biochemical and morphological changes
- Abnormalities accumulate as tumour progresses
- See cancer genes map

Tumour angiogenesis
- Oxygen and nutrition required
- Tumour angiogenesis factors (TAF)
  - Vascular endothelial growth factor (vegf)
  - Fibroblast growth factor (fgf)
- Antiangiogenesis factors
  - Angiostatin
  - Endostatin

Differentiation
- Well differentiated resembles normal tissue
- May lose differentiation as tumour progresses
- Poorly differentiated resembles embryonic tissue
- Well differentiated - often low grade poorly differentiated - often high grade

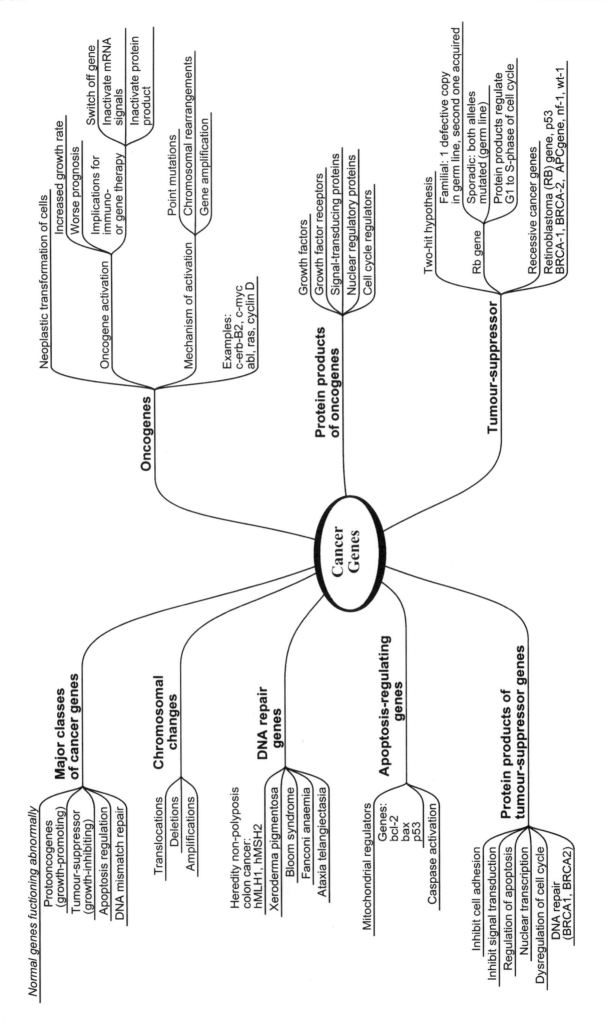

GENERAL PATHOLOGY

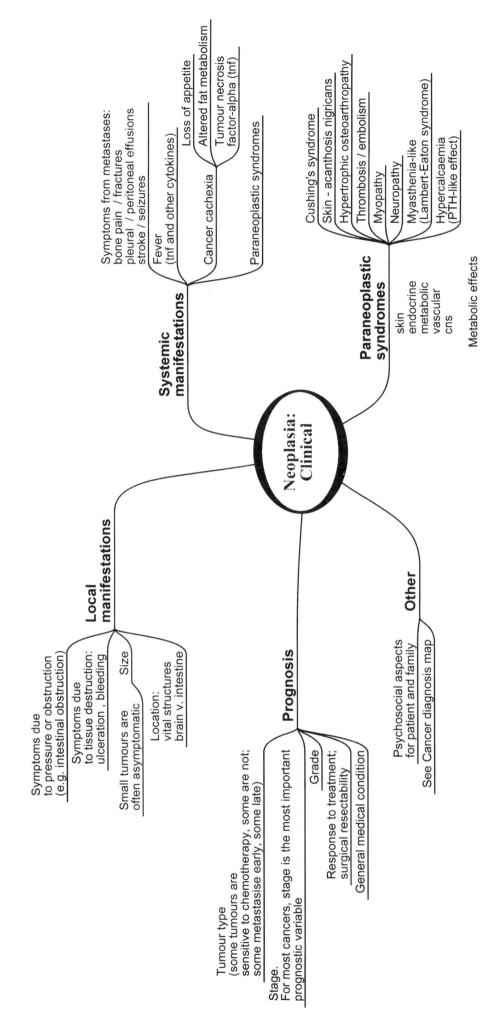

Neoplasia: Clinical

Systemic manifestations

Symptoms from metastases: bone pain / fractures pleural / peritoneal effusions stroke / seizures

Fever (tnf and other cytokines)

Loss of appetite
Altered fat metabolism
Tumour necrosis factor-alpha (tnf)

Cancer cachexia

Paraneoplastic syndromes

Paraneoplastic syndromes

Cushing's syndrome
Skin - acanthosis nigricans
Hypertrophic osteoarthropathy
Thrombosis / embolism
Myopathy
Neuropathy
Myasthenia-like (Lambert-Eaton syndrome)
Hypercalcaemia (PTH-like effect)

skin
endocrine
metabolic
vascular
cns

Metabolic effects

Local manifestations

Symptoms due to pressure or obstruction (e.g. intestinal obstruction)

Symptoms due to tissue destruction: ulceration , bleeding

Size

Small tumours are often asymptomatic

Location: vital structures brain v. intestine

Prognosis

Tumour type (some tumours are sensitive to chemotherapy, some are not; some metastasise early, some late)

Stage. For most cancers, stage is the most important prognostic variable

Grade

Response to treatment; surgical resectability

General medical condition

Other

Psychosocial aspects for patient and family

See Cancer diagnosis map

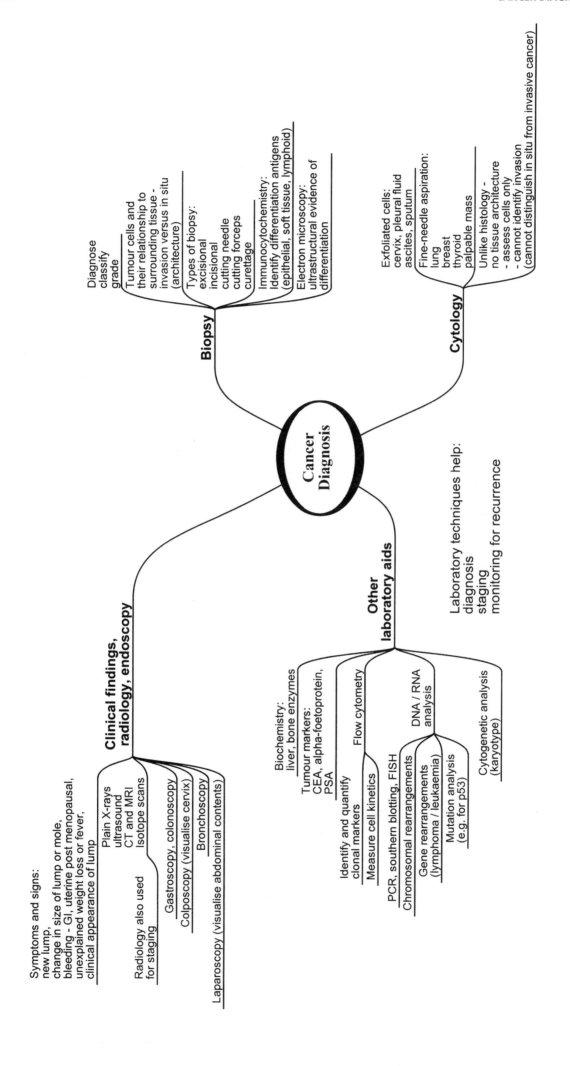

Cancer Diagnosis

Clinical findings, radiology, endoscopy

Symptoms and signs:
new lump,
change in size of lump or mole,
bleeding - GI, uterine post menopausal,
unexplained weight loss or fever,
clinical appearance of lump

Plain X-rays
ultrasound
CT and MRI
Isotope scans

Radiology also used for staging

Gastroscopy, colonoscopy
Colposcopy (visualise cervix)
Bronchoscopy

Laparoscopy (visualise abdominal contents)

Biopsy

Diagnose
classify
grade

Tumour cells and their relationship to surrounding tissue - invasion versus in situ (architecture)

Types of biopsy:
excisional
incisional
cutting needle
cutting forceps
curettage

Immunocytochemistry:
Identify differentiation antigens (epithelial, soft tissue, lymphoid)

Electron microscopy:
ultrastructural evidence of differentiation

Cytology

Exfoliated cells:
cervix, pleural fluid
ascites, sputum

Fine-needle aspiration:
lung
breast
thyroid
palpable mass

Unlike histology -
no tissue architecture
- assess cells only
- cannot identify invasion
(cannot distinguish in situ from invasive cancer)

Other laboratory aids

Biochemistry:
liver, bone enzymes

Tumour markers:
CEA, alpha-foetoprotein, PSA

Flow cytometry

Identify and quantify clonal markers

Measure cell kinetics

PCR, southern blotting, FISH
Chromosomal rearrangements

DNA / RNA analysis

Gene rearrangements (lymphoma / leukaemia)

Mutation analysis (e.g. for p53)

Cytogenetic analysis (karyotype)

Laboratory techniques help:
diagnosis
staging
monitoring for recurrence

DISEASES OF INFANCY AND CHILDHOOD

SYSTEMIC PATHOLOGY

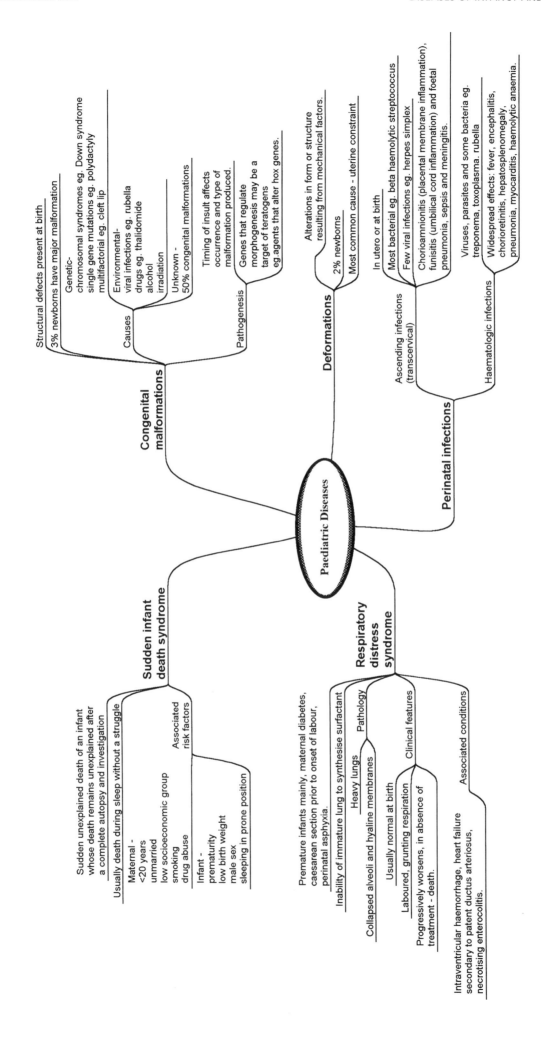

Paediatric Diseases

Congenital malformations

Structural defects present at birth
3% newborns have major malformation

Causes

- Genetic-
chromosomal syndromes eg. Down syndrome
single gene mutations eg. polydactyly
multifactorial eg. cleft lip

- Environmental-
viral infections eg. rubella
drugs eg. thalidomide
alcohol
irradiation

- Unknown -
50% congenital malformations

Pathogenesis

- Timing of insult affects occurrence and type of malformation produced.

- Genes that regulate morphogenesis may be a target of teratogens eg. agents that alter hox genes.

Deformations

- Alterations in form or structure resulting from mechanical factors.

- 2% newborns

- Most common cause - uterine constraint

Perinatal infections

- In utero or at birth

Ascending infections (transcervical)

- Most bacterial eg. beta haemolytic streptococcus
- Few viral infections eg. herpes simplex
- Chorioamnionitis (placental membrane inflammation), funisitis (umbilical cord inflammation) and foetal pneumonia, sepsis and meningitis.

Haematologic infections

- Viruses, parasites and some bacteria eg. treponema, toxoplasma. rubella
- Widespread effects: fever, encephalitis, chorioretinitis, hepatosplenomegaly, pneumonia, myocarditis, haemolytic anaemia.

Sudden infant death syndrome

Sudden unexplained death of an infant whose death remains unexplained after a complete autopsy and investigation

Usually death during sleep without a struggle

Associated risk factors

- Maternal -
<20 years
unmarried
low socioeconomic group
smoking
drug abuse

- Infant -
prematurity
low birth weight
male sex
sleeping in prone position

Respiratory distress syndrome

Premature infants mainly, maternal diabetes, caesarean section prior to onset of labour, perinatal asphyxia.

Inability of immature lung to synthesise surfactant

Pathology

- Heavy lungs
- Collapsed alveoli and hyaline membranes

Clinical features

- Usually normal at birth
- Laboured, grunting respiration
- Progressively worsens, in absence of treatment - death.

Associated conditions

- Intraventricular haemorrhage, heart failure secondary to patent ductus arteriosus, necrotising enterocolitis.

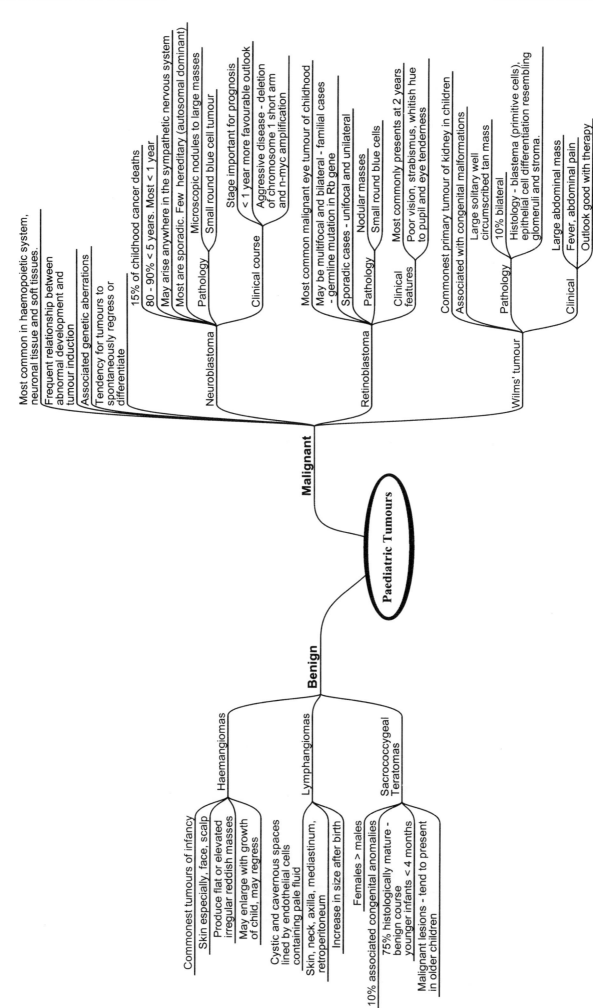

Paediatric Tumours

Malignant

Neuroblastoma

- Most common in haemopoietic system, neuronal tissue and soft tissues.
- Frequent relationship between abnormal development and tumour induction
- Associated genetic aberrations
- Tendency for tumours to spontaneously regress or differentiate
- 15% of childhood cancer deaths
- 80 - 90% < 5 years. Most < 1 year
- May arise anywhere in the sympathetic nervous system
- Most are sporadic. Few hereditary (autosomal dominant)

Pathology
- Microscopic nodules to large masses
- Small round blue cell tumour

Clinical course
- Stage important for prognosis
- < 1 year more favourable outlook
- Aggressive disease - deletion of chromosome 1 short arm and n-myc amplification

Retinoblastoma

- Most common malignant eye tumour of childhood
- May be multifocal and bilateral - familial cases - germline mutation in Rb gene
- Sporadic cases - unifocal and unilateral

Pathology
- Nodular masses
- Small round blue cells

Clinical features
- Most commonly presents at 2 years
- Poor vision, strabismus, whitish hue to pupil and eye tenderness

Wilms' tumour

- Commonest primary tumour of kidney in children
- Associated with congenital malformations

Pathology
- Large solitary well circumscribed tan mass
- 10% bilateral
- Histology - blastema (primitive cells), epithelial cell differentiation resembling glomeruli and stroma.

Clinical
- Large abdominal mass
- Fever, abdominal pain
- Outlook good with therapy

Benign

Haemangiomas
- Commonest tumours of infancy
- Skin especially, face, scalp
- Produce flat or elevated irregular reddish masses
- May enlarge with growth of child, may regress

Lymphangiomas
- Cystic and cavernous spaces lined by endothelial cells containing pale fluid
- Skin, neck, axilla, mediastinum, retroperitoneum
- Increase in size after birth

Sacrococcygeal Teratomas
- Females > males
- 10% associated congenital anomalies
- 75% histologically mature - benign course younger infants < 4 months
- Malignant lesions - tend to present in older children

CARDIO-VASCULAR SYSTEM

SYSTEMATIC PATHOLOGY

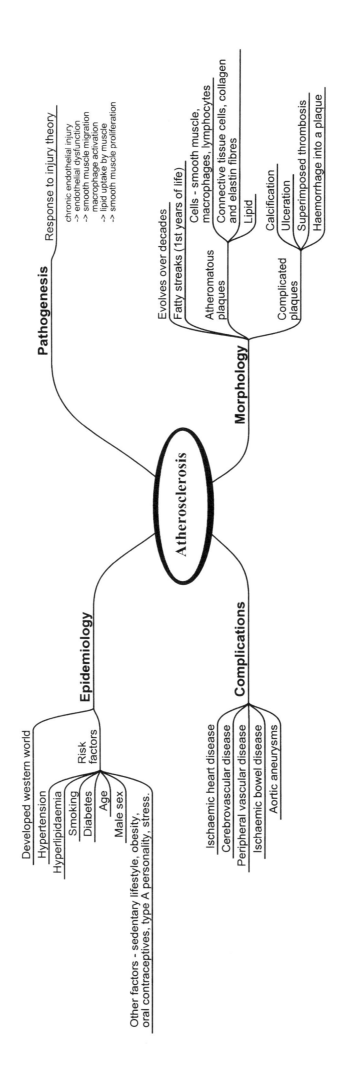

Atherosclerosis

Pathogenesis

Response to injury theory

chronic endothelial injury
-> endothelial dysfunction
-> smooth muscle migration
-> macrophage activation
-> lipid uptake by muscle
-> smooth muscle proliferation

Morphology

Evolves over decades

Fatty streaks (1st years of life)

Atheromatous plaques

Cells - smooth muscle, macrophages, lymphocytes

Connective tissue cells, collagen and elastin fibres

Lipid

Complicated plaques

Calcification

Ulceration

Superimposed thrombosis

Haemorrhage into a plaque

Epidemiology

Developed western world

Hypertension

Hyperlipidaemia

Smoking

Diabetes

Age

Male sex

Risk factors

Other factors - sedentary lifestyle, obesity, oral contraceptives, type A personality, stress.

Complications

Ischaemic heart disease

Cerebrovascular disease

Peripheral vascular disease

Ischaemic bowel disease

Aortic aneurysms

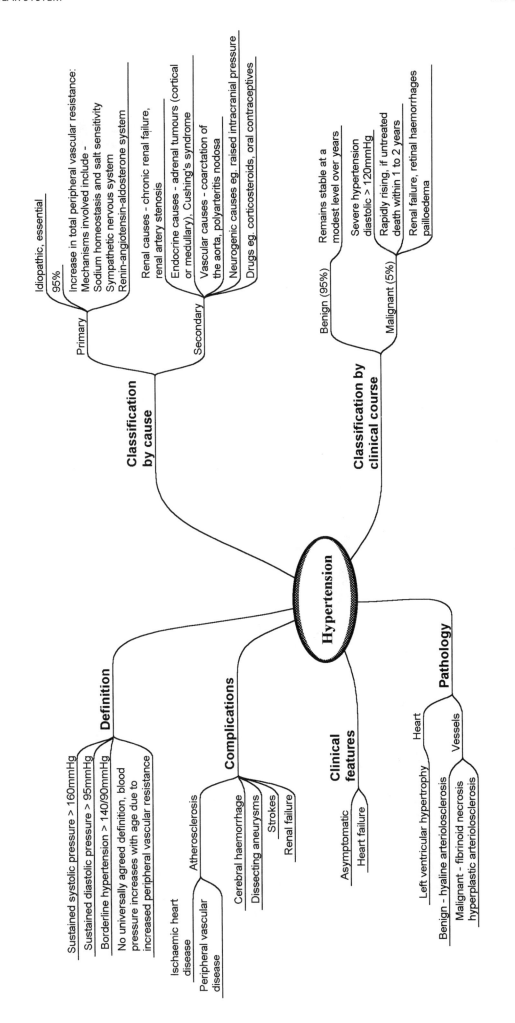

Classification by cause

Primary

Idiopathic, essential

95%

Increase in total peripheral vascular resistance:
Mechanisms involved include -
Sodium homeostasis and salt sensitivity
Sympathetic nervous system
Renin-angiotensin-aldosterone system

Secondary

Renal causes - chronic renal failure,
renal artery stenosis

Endocrine causes - adrenal tumours (cortical
or medullary), Cushing's syndrome

Vascular causes - coarctation of
the aorta, polyarteritis nodosa

Neurogenic causes eg. raised intracranial pressure

Drugs eg. corticosteroids, oral contraceptives

Classification by clinical course

Benign (95%)

Remains stable at a
modest level over years

Malignant (5%)

Severe hypertension
diastolic > 120mmHg

Rapidly rising, if untreated
death within 1 to 2 years

Renal failure, retinal haemorrhages
pailloedema

Hypertension

Definition

Sustained systolic pressure > 160mmHg

Sustained diastolic pressure > 95mmHg

Borderline hypertension > 140/90mmHg

No universally agreed definition, blood
pressure increases with age due to
increased peripheral vascular resistance

Complications

Ischaemic heart
disease

Atherosclerosis

Peripheral vascular
disease

Cerebral haemorrhage

Dissecting aneurysms

Strokes

Renal failure

Clinical features

Asymptomatic

Heart failure

Pathology

Heart

Left ventricular hypertrophy

Vessels

Benign - hyaline arteriolosclerosis

Malignant - fibrinoid necrosis
hyperplastic arteriolosclerosis

SYSTEMATIC PATHOLOGY

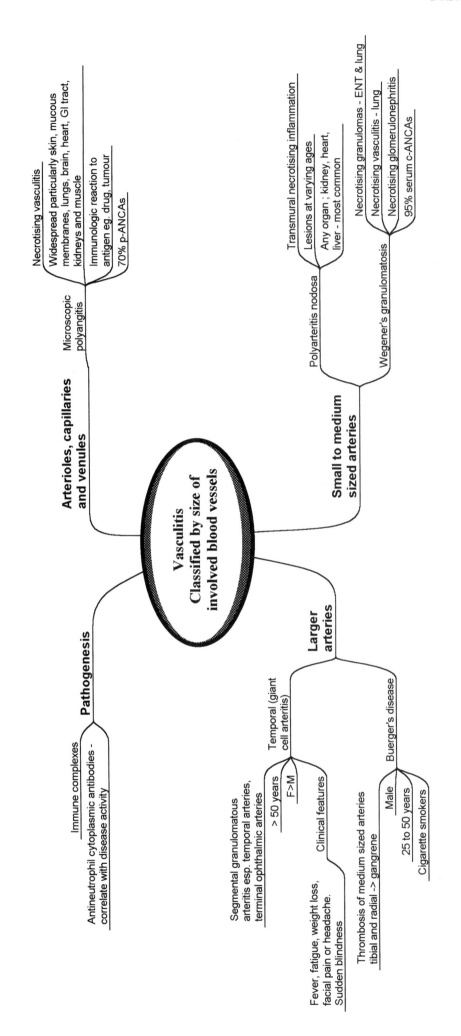

Vasculitis
Classified by size of involved blood vessels

Arterioles, capillaries and venules

Microscopic polyangitis

Necrotising vasculitis

Widespread particularly skin, mucous membranes, lungs, brain, heart, GI tract, kidneys and muscle

Immunologic reaction to antigen eg. drug, tumour

70% p-ANCAs

Small to medium sized arteries

Polyarteritis nodosa

Transmural necrotising inflammation

Lesions at varying ages

Any organ ; kidney, heart, liver - most common

Wegener's granulomatosis

Necrotising granulomas - ENT & lung

Necrotising vasculitis - lung

Necrotising glomerulonephritis

95% serum c-ANCAs

Pathogenesis

Immune complexes

Antineutrophil cytoplasmic antibodies - correlate with disease activity

Larger arteries

Temporal (giant cell arteritis)

Segmental granulomatous arteritis esp. temporal arteries, terminal ophthalmic arteries

> 50 years

F>M

Clinical features

Fever, fatigue, weight loss, facial pain or headache. Sudden blindness

Buerger's disease

Thrombosis of medium sized arteries tibial and radial -> gangrene

Male

25 to 50 years

Cigarette smokers

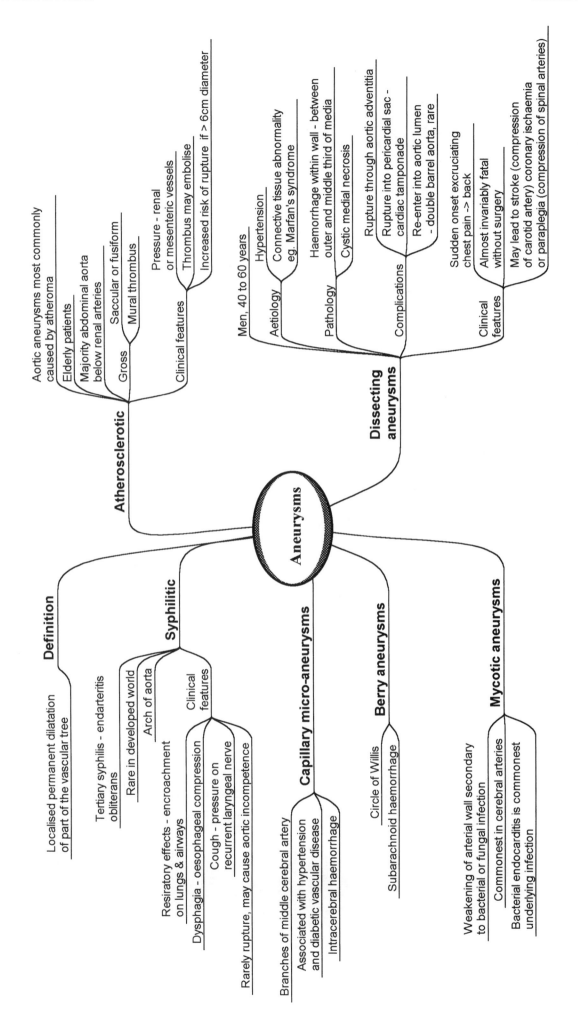

Aneurysms

Definition
- Localised permanent dilatation of part of the vascular tree

Atherosclerotic
- Aortic aneurysms most commonly caused by atheroma
- Elderly patients
- Majority abdominal aorta below renal arteries
- Gross
  - Saccular or fusiform
  - Mural thrombus
- Clinical features
  - Pressure - renal or mesenteric vessels
  - Thrombus may embolise
  - Increased risk of rupture if > 6cm diameter

Dissecting aneurysms
- Men, 40 to 60 years
- Aetiology
  - Hypertension
  - Connective tissue abnormality eg. Marfan's syndrome
- Pathology
  - Haemorrhage within wall - between outer and middle third of media
  - Cystic medial necrosis
- Complications
  - Rupture through aortic adventitia
  - Rupture into pericardial sac - cardiac tamponade
  - Re-enter into aortic lumen - double barrel aorta, rare
- Clinical features
  - Sudden onset excruciating chest pain -> back
  - Almost invariably fatal without surgery
  - May lead to stroke (compression of carotid artery) coronary ischaemia or paraplegia (compression of spinal arteries)

Syphilitic
- Tertiary syphilis - endarteritis obliterans
- Rare in developed world
- Arch of aorta
- Clinical features
  - Resiratory effects - encroachment on lungs & airways
  - Dysphagia - oesophageal compression
  - Cough - pressure on recurrent laryngeal nerve
  - Rarely rupture, may cause aortic incompetence

Capillary micro-aneurysms
- Branches of middle cerebral artery
- Associated with hypertension and diabetic vascular disease
- Intracerebral haemorrhage

Berry aneurysms
- Circle of Willis
- Subarachnoid haemorrhage

Mycotic aneurysms
- Weakening of arterial wall secondary to bacterial or fungal infection
- Commonest in cerebral arteries
- Bacterial endocarditis is commonest underlying infection

SYSTEMATIC PATHOLOGY

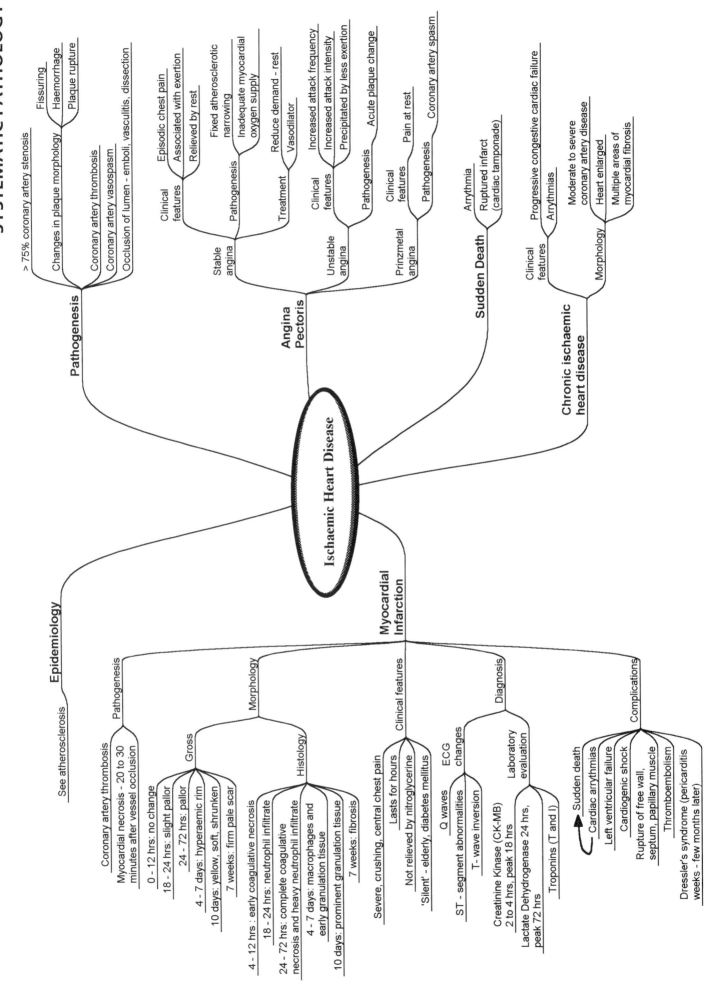

Ischaemic Heart Disease

Pathogenesis

> 75% coronary artery stenosis

Changes in plaque morphology
- Fissuring
- Haemorrhage
- Plaque rupture

Coronary artery thrombosis
Coronary artery vasospasm
Occlusion of lumen – emboli, vasculitis, dissection

Angina Pectoris

Stable angina
- Clinical features
  - Episodic chest pain
  - Associated with exertion
  - Relieved by rest
- Pathogenesis
  - Fixed atherosclerotic narrowing
  - Inadequate myocardial oxygen supply
- Treatment
  - Reduce demand - rest
  - Vasodilator

Unstable angina
- Clinical features
  - Increased attack frequency
  - Increased attack intensity
  - Precipitated by less exertion
- Pathogenesis
  - Acute plaque change

Prinzmetal angina
- Clinical features
  - Pain at rest
- Pathogenesis
  - Coronary artery spasm

Sudden Death

Arrythmia
Ruptured infarct (cardiac tamponade)

Chronic ischaemic heart disease

Clinical features
- Progressive congestive cardiac failure
- Arrythmias

Morphology
- Moderate to severe coronary artery disease
- Heart enlarged
- Multiple areas of myocardial fibrosis

Epidemiology

See atherosclerosis

Myocardial Infarction

Pathogenesis
- Coronary artery thrombosis
- Myocardial necrosis - 20 to 30 minutes after vessel occlusion

Morphology
- Gross
  - 0 - 12 hrs: no change
  - 18 - 24 hrs: slight pallor
  - 24 - 72 hrs: pallor
  - 4 - 7 days: hyperaemic rim
  - 10 days: yellow, soft, shrunken
  - 7 weeks: firm pale scar
- Histology
  - 4 - 12 hrs : early coagulative necrosis
  - 18 - 24 hrs: neutrophil infiltrate
  - 24 - 72 hrs: complete coagulative necrosis and heavy neutrophil infiltrate
  - 4 - 7 days: macrophages and early granulation tissue
  - 10 days: prominent granulation tissue
  - 7 weeks: fibrosis

Clinical features
- Severe, crushing, central chest pain
- Lasts for hours
- Not relieved by nitroglycerine
- 'Silent' - elderly, diabetes mellitus

Diagnosis
- ECG changes
  - Q waves
  - ST - segment abnormalities
  - T- wave inversion
- Laboratory evaluation
  - Creatinine Kinase (CK-MB) 2 to 4 hrs, peak 18 hrs
  - Lactate Dehydrogenase 24 hrs, peak 72 hrs
  - Troponins (T and I)

Complications
- Sudden death
- Cardiac arrythmias
- Left ventricular failure
- Cardiogenic shock
- Rupture of free wall, septum, papillary muscle
- Thromboembolism
- Dressler's syndrome (pericarditis weeks - few months later)

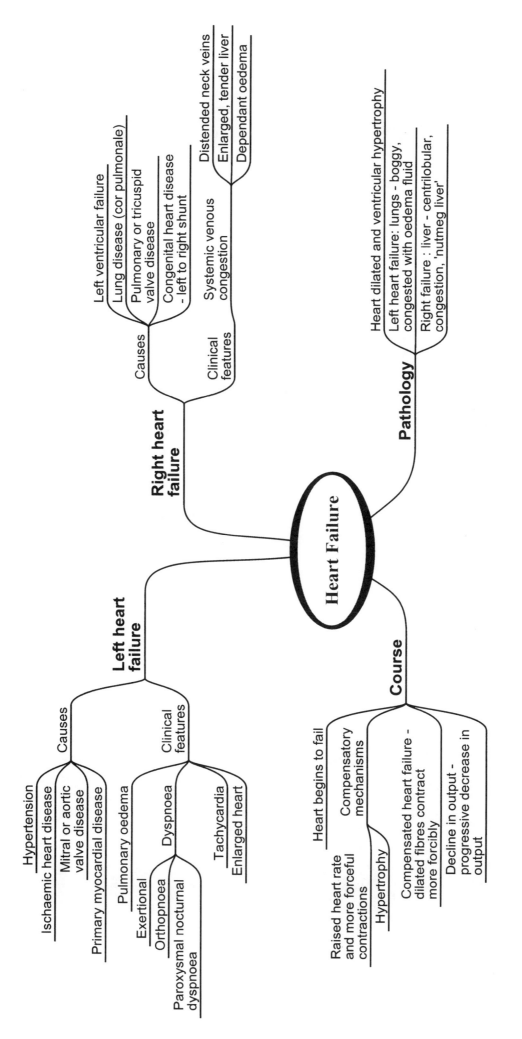

Heart Failure

Right heart failure

Causes
- Left ventricular failure
- Lung disease (cor pulmonale)
- Pulmonary or tricuspid valve disease
- Congenital heart disease - left to right shunt

Clinical features
- Systemic venous congestion
  - Distended neck veins
  - Enlarged, tender liver
  - Dependant oedema

Pathology
- Heart dilated and ventricular hypertrophy
- Left heart failure: lungs - boggy, congested with oedema fluid
- Right failure : liver - centrilobular, congestion, 'nutmeg liver'

Left heart failure

Causes
- Hypertension
- Ischaemic heart disease
- Mitral or aortic valve disease
- Primary myocardial disease

Clinical features
- Pulmonary oedema
- Dyspnoea
  - Exertional
  - Orthopnoea
  - Paroxysmal nocturnal dyspnoea
- Tachycardia
- Enlarged heart

Course
- Heart begins to fail
- Compensatory mechanisms
  - Raised heart rate and more forceful contractions
  - Hypertrophy
- Compensated heart failure - dilated fibres contract more forcibly
- Decline in output - progressive decrease in output

SYSTEMATIC PATHOLOGY

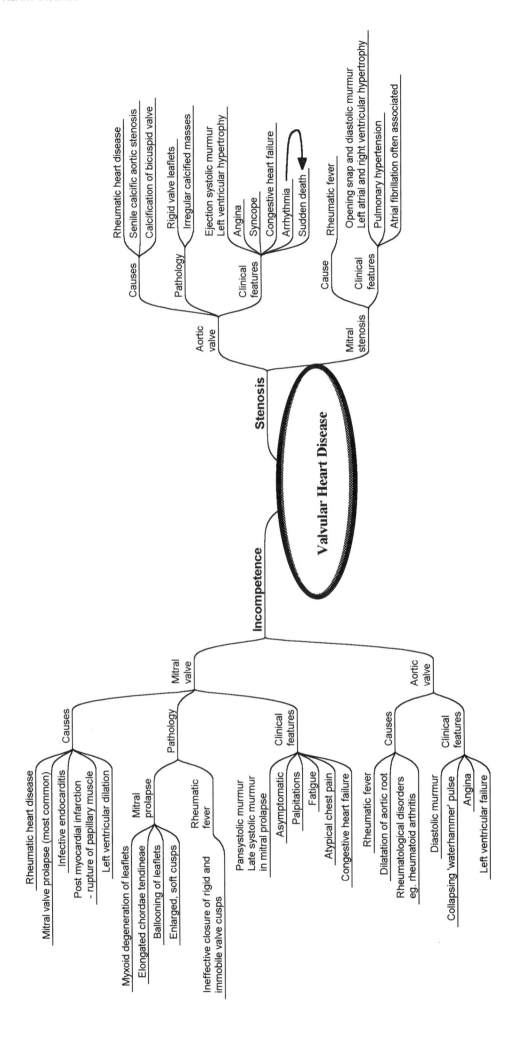

Valvular Heart Disease

Stenosis

Aortic valve

Causes
- Rheumatic heart disease
- Senile calcific aortic stenosis
- Calcification of bicuspid valve

Pathology
- Rigid valve leaflets
- Irregular calcified masses

Clinical features
- Ejection systolic murmur
- Left ventricular hypertrophy
- Angina
- Syncope
- Congestive heart failure
- Arrhythmia
- Sudden death

Mitral stenosis

Cause
- Rheumatic fever

Clinical features
- Opening snap and diastolic murmur
- Left atrial and right ventricular hypertrophy
- Pulmonary hypertension
- Atrial fibrillation often associated

Incompetence

Mitral valve

Causes
- Rheumatic heart disease
- Mitral valve prolapse (most common)
- Infective endocarditis
- Post myocardial infarction
  - rupture of papillary muscle
- Left ventricular dilation

Mitral prolapse
- Myxoid degeneration of leaflets
- Elongated chordae tendineae
- Ballooning of leaflets
- Enlarged, soft cusps

Pathology

Rheumatic fever
- Ineffective closure of rigid and immobile valve cusps

Clinical features
- Pansystolic murmur
- Late systolic murmur in mitral prolapse
- Asymptomatic
- Palpitations
- Fatigue
- Atypical chest pain
- Congestive heart failure

Aortic valve

Causes
- Rheumatic fever
- Dilatation of aortic root
- Rheumatological disorders eg. rheumatoid arthritis

Clinical features
- Diastolic murmur
- Collapsing 'waterhammer' pulse
- Angina
- Left ventricular failure

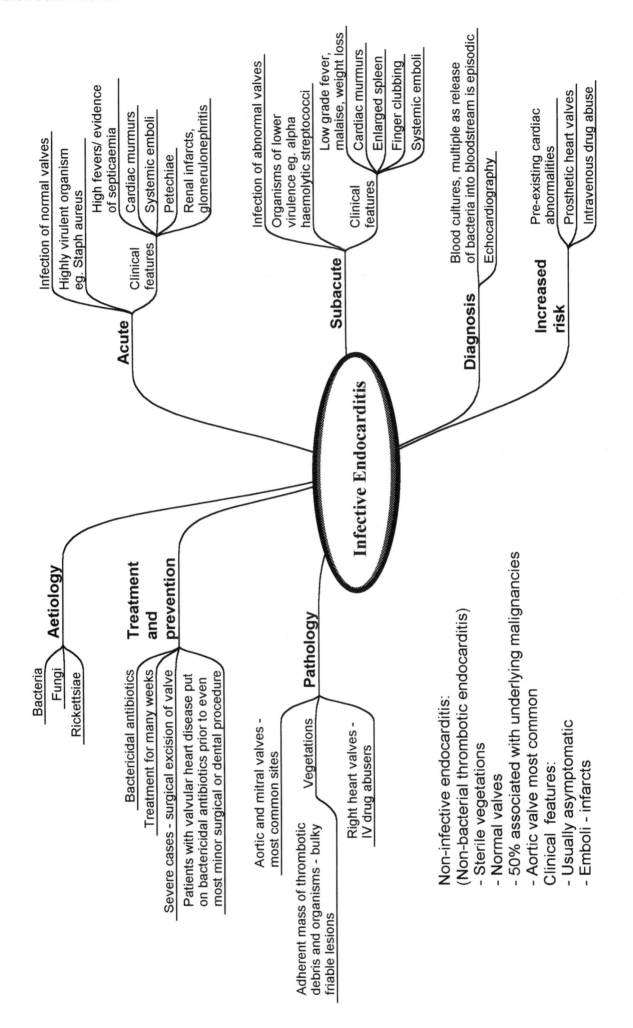

Infective Endocarditis

Acute

Infection of normal valves

Highly virulent organism eg. Staph aureus

High fevers/ evidence of septicaemia

Clinical features
- Cardiac murmurs
- Systemic emboli
- Petechiae
- Renal infarcts, glomerulonephritis

Subacute

Infection of abnormal valves

Organisms of lower virulence eg. alpha haemolytic streptococci

Low grade fever, malaise, weight loss

Clinical features
- Cardiac murmurs
- Enlarged spleen
- Finger clubbing
- Systemic emboli

Diagnosis

Blood cultures, multiple as release of bacteria into bloodstream is episodic

Echocardiography

Increased risk

Pre-existing cardiac abnormalities

Prosthetic heart valves

Intravenous drug abuse

Aetiology

Bacteria

Fungi

Rickettsiae

Treatment and prevention

Bactericidal antibiotics

Treatment for many weeks

Severe cases - surgical excision of valve

Patients with valvular heart disease put on bactericidal antibiotics prior to even most minor surgical or dental procedure

Pathology

Aortic and mitral valves - most common sites

Vegetations

Adherent mass of thrombotic debris and organisms - bulky friable lesions

Right heart valves - IV drug abusers

Non-infective endocarditis:
(Non-bacterial thrombotic endocarditis)
- Sterile vegetations
- Normal valves
- 50% associated with underlying malignancies
- Aortic valve most common
Clinical features:
- Usually asymptomatic
- Emboli - infarcts

SYSTEMATIC PATHOLOGY

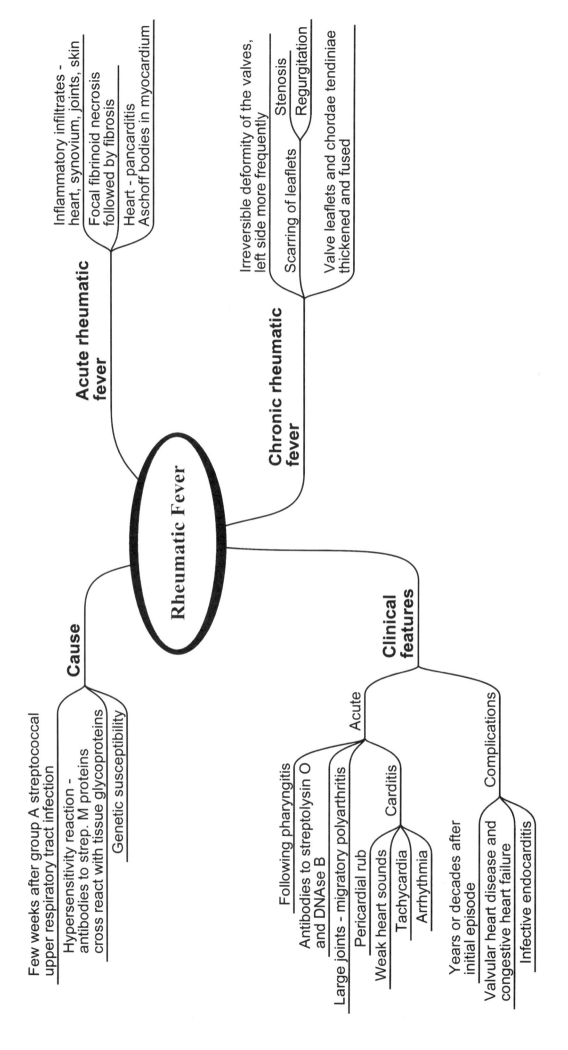

Rheumatic Fever

Acute rheumatic fever

Inflammatory infiltrates - heart, synovium, joints, skin

Focal fibrinoid necrosis followed by fibrosis

Heart - pancarditis
Aschoff bodies in myocardium

Chronic rheumatic fever

Irreversible deformity of the valves, left side more frequently

Scarring of leaflets

Stenosis

Regurgitation

Valve leaflets and chordae tendiniae thickened and fused

Cause

Few weeks after group A streptococcal upper respiratory tract infection

Hypersensitivity reaction - antibodies to strep. M proteins cross react with tissue glycoproteins

Genetic susceptibility

Clinical features

Acute

Following pharyngitis

Antibodies to streptolysin O and DNAse B

Large joints - migratory polyarthritis

Pericardial rub

Weak heart sounds

Carditis

Tachycardia

Arrhythmia

Complications

Years or decades after initial episode

Valvular heart disease and congestive heart failure

Infective endocarditis

SYSTEMATIC PATHOLOGY

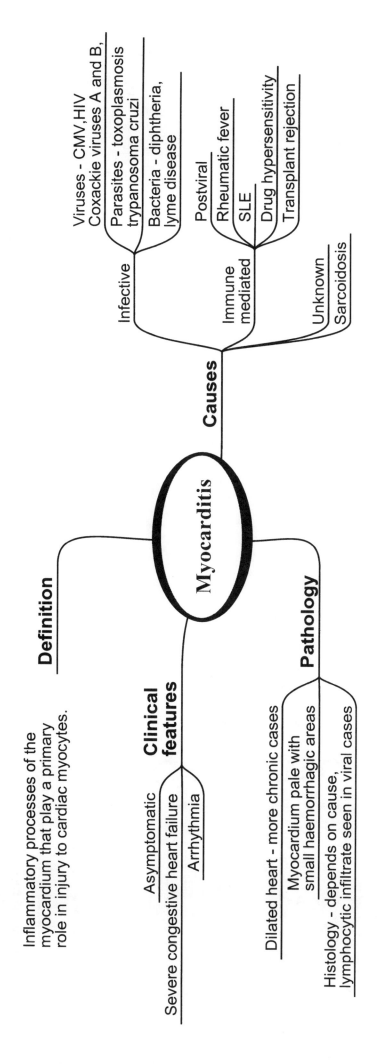

Myocarditis

Definition

Inflammatory processes of the myocardium that play a primary role in injury to cardiac myocytes.

Causes

Infective
- Viruses - CMV, HIV Coxackie viruses A and B,
- Parasites - toxoplasmosis trypanosoma cruzi
- Bacteria - diphtheria, lyme disease

Immune mediated
- Postviral
- Rheumatic fever
- SLE
- Drug hypersensitivity
- Transplant rejection

Unknown
- Sarcoidosis

Clinical features
- Asymptomatic
- Severe congestive heart failure
- Arrhythmia

Pathology
- Dilated heart - more chronic cases
- Myocardium pale with small haemorrhagic areas
- Histology - depends on cause, lymphocytic infiltrate seen in viral cases

SYSTEMATIC PATHOLOGY

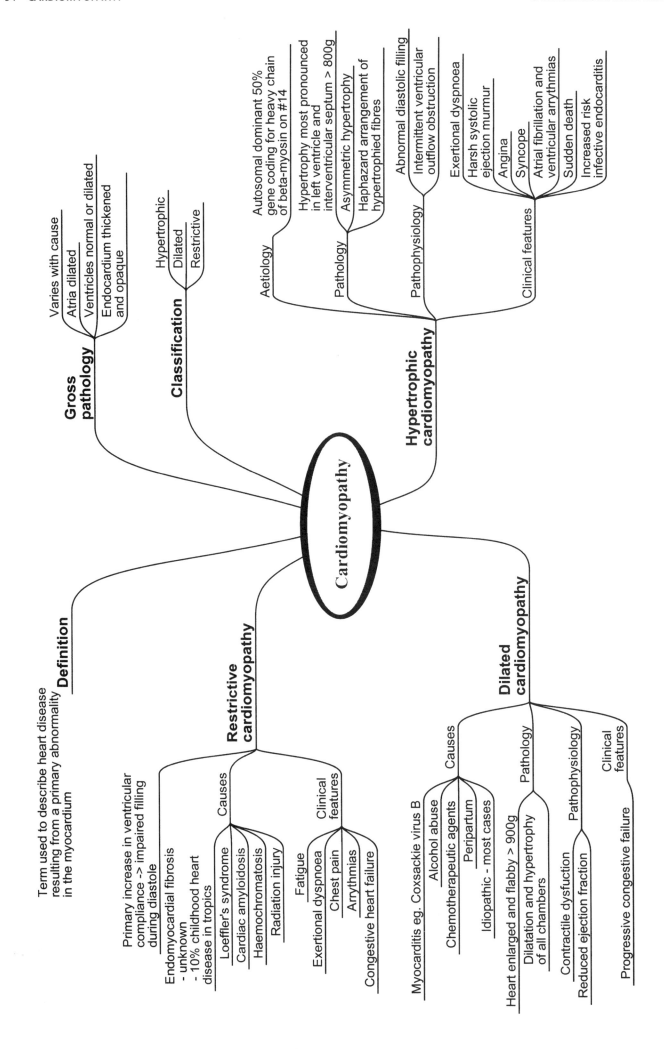

Cardiomyopathy

Definition
Term used to describe heart disease resulting from a primary abnormality in the myocardium

Gross pathology
- Varies with cause
- Atria dilated
- Ventricles normal or dilated
- Endocardium thickened and opaque

Classification
- Hypertrophic
- Dilated
- Restrictive

Hypertrophic cardiomyopathy

Aetiology
- Autosomal dominant 50% gene coding for heavy chain of beta-myosin on #14

Pathology
- Hypertrophy most pronounced in left ventricle and interventricular septum > 800g
- Asymmetric hypertrophy
- Haphazard arrangement of hypertrophied fibres

Pathophysiology
- Abnormal diastolic filling
- Intermittent ventricular outflow obstruction

Clinical features
- Exertional dyspnoea
- Harsh systolic ejection murmur
- Angina
- Syncope
- Atrial fibrillation and ventricular arrythmias
- Sudden death
- Increased risk infective endocarditis

Restrictive cardiomyopathy

Causes
- Endomyocardial fibrosis
  - unknown
  - 10% childhood heart disease in tropics
- Loeffler's syndrome
- Cardiac amyloidosis
- Haemochromatosis
- Radiation injury

Primary increase in ventricular compliance -> impaired filling during diastole

Clinical features
- Fatigue
- Exertional dyspnoea
- Chest pain
- Arrythmias
- Congestive heart failure

Dilated cardiomyopathy

Causes
- Myocarditis eg. Coxsackie virus B
- Alcohol abuse
- Chemotherapeutic agents
- Peripartum
- Idiopathic - most cases

Pathology
- Heart enlarged and flabby > 900g
- Dilatation and hypertrophy of all chambers

Pathophysiology
- Contractile dysfuction
- Reduced ejection fraction

Clinical features
- Progressive congestive failure

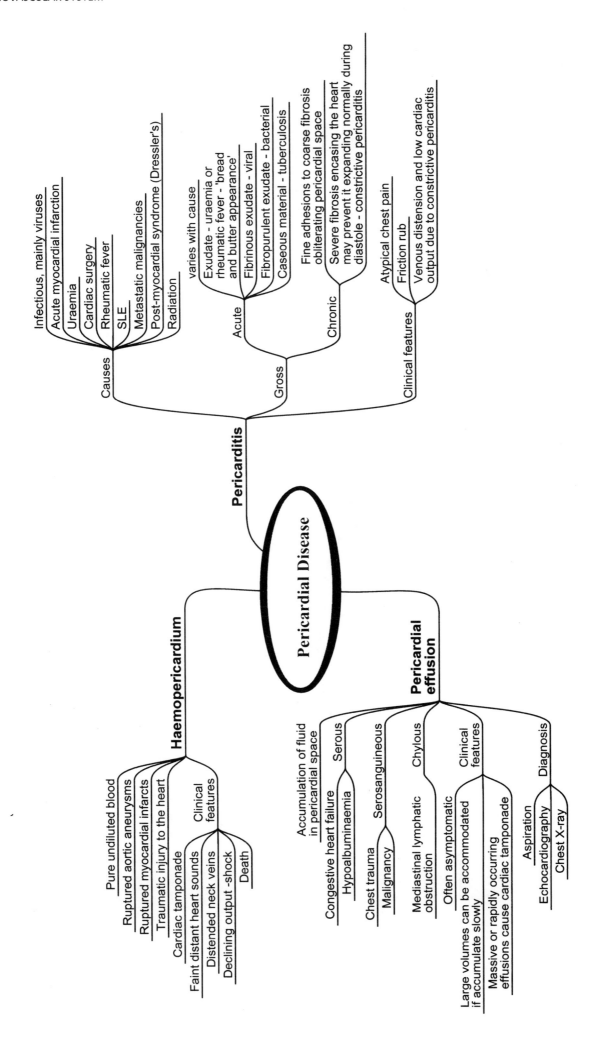

Pericardial Disease

Pericarditis

Causes
- Infectious, mainly viruses
- Acute myocardial infarction
- Uraemia
- Cardiac surgery
- Rheumatic fever
- SLE
- Metastatic malignancies
- Post-myocardial syndrome (Dressler's)
- Radiation

Gross
- Acute — varies with cause
  - Exudate - uraemia or rheumatic fever - 'bread and butter appearance'
  - Fibrinous exudate - viral
  - Fibropurulent exudate - bacterial
  - Caseous material - tuberculosis
- Chronic
  - Fine adhesions to coarse fibrosis obliterating pericardial space
  - Severe fibrosis encasing the heart may prevent it expanding normally during diastole - constrictive pericarditis

Clinical features
- Atypical chest pain
- Friction rub
- Venous distension and low cardiac output due to constrictive pericarditis

Haemopericardium
- Pure undiluted blood
- Ruptured aortic aneurysms
- Ruptured myocardial infarcts
- Traumatic injury to the heart
- Cardiac tamponade
- Clinical features
  - Faint distant heart sounds
  - Distended neck veins
  - Declining output -shock
  - Death

Pericardial effusion
- Accumulation of fluid in pericardial space
- Serous
  - Congestive heart failure
  - Hypoalbuminaemia
- Serosanguineous
  - Chest trauma
  - Malignancy
- Chylous
  - Mediastinal lymphatic obstruction
- Clinical features
  - Often asymptomatic
  - Large volumes can be accommodated if accumulate slowly
  - Massive or rapidly occurring effusions cause cardiac tamponade
- Diagnosis
  - Aspiration
  - Echocardiography
  - Chest X-ray

SYSTEMATIC PATHOLOGY

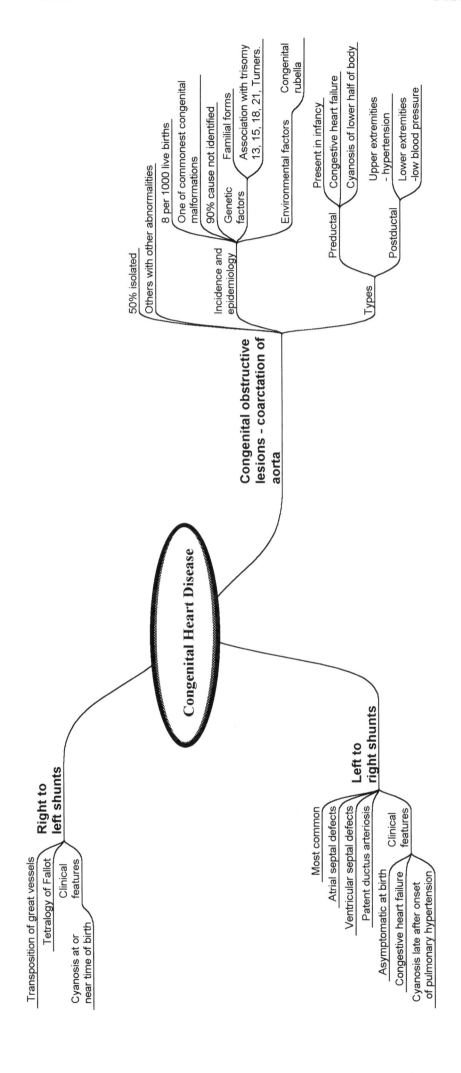

Congenital Heart Disease

Congenital obstructive lesions - coarctation of aorta

Incidence and epidemiology
- 50% isolated
- Others with other abnormalities
- 8 per 1000 live births
- One of commonest congenital malformations
- 90% cause not identified
- Genetic factors
  - Familial forms
  - Association with trisomy 13, 15, 18, 21, Turners.
- Environmental factors
  - Congenital rubella

Types
- Preductal
  - Present in infancy
  - Congestive heart failure
  - Cyanosis of lower half of body
- Postductal
  - Upper extremities - hypertension
  - Lower extremities -low blood pressure

Right to left shunts
- Transposition of great vessels
- Tetralogy of Fallot
- Clinical features
  - Cyanosis at or near time of birth

Left to right shunts
- Most common
- Atrial septal defects
- Ventricular septal defects
- Patent ductus arteriosis
- Clinical features
  - Asymptomatic at birth
  - Congestive heart failure
  - Cyanosis late after onset of pulmonary hypertension

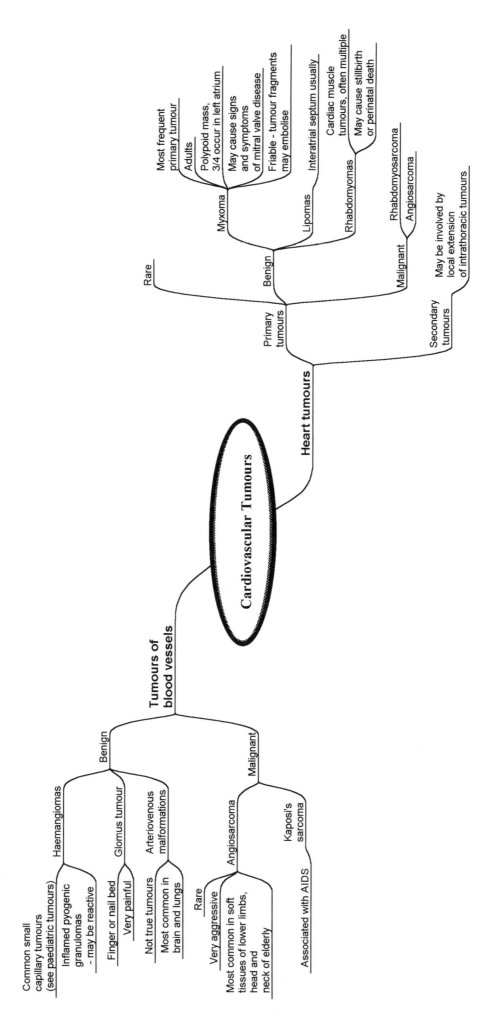

Cardiovascular Tumours

Heart tumours

Primary tumours

Rare

Benign

Myxoma
- Most frequent primary tumour
- Adults
- Polypoid mass, 3/4 occur in left atrium
- May cause signs and symptoms of mitral valve disease
- Friable - tumour fragments may embolise

Lipomas
- Interatrial septum usually

Rhabdomyomas
- Cardiac muscle tumours, often multiple
- May cause stillbirth or perinatal death

Malignant
- Rhabdomyosarcoma
- Angiosarcoma

Secondary tumours
- May be involved by local extension of intrathoracic tumours

Tumours of blood vessels

Benign

Haemangiomas
- Common small capillary tumours (see paediatric tumours)
- Inflamed pyogenic granulomas - may be reactive

Glomus tumour
- Finger or nail bed
- Very painful

Arteriovenous malformations
- Not true tumours
- Most common in brain and lungs
- Rare

Malignant

Angiosarcoma
- Very aggressive
- Most common in soft tissues of lower limbs, head and neck of elderly

Kaposi's sarcoma
- Associated with AIDS

RESPIRATORY TRACT

SYSTEMATIC PATHOLOGY

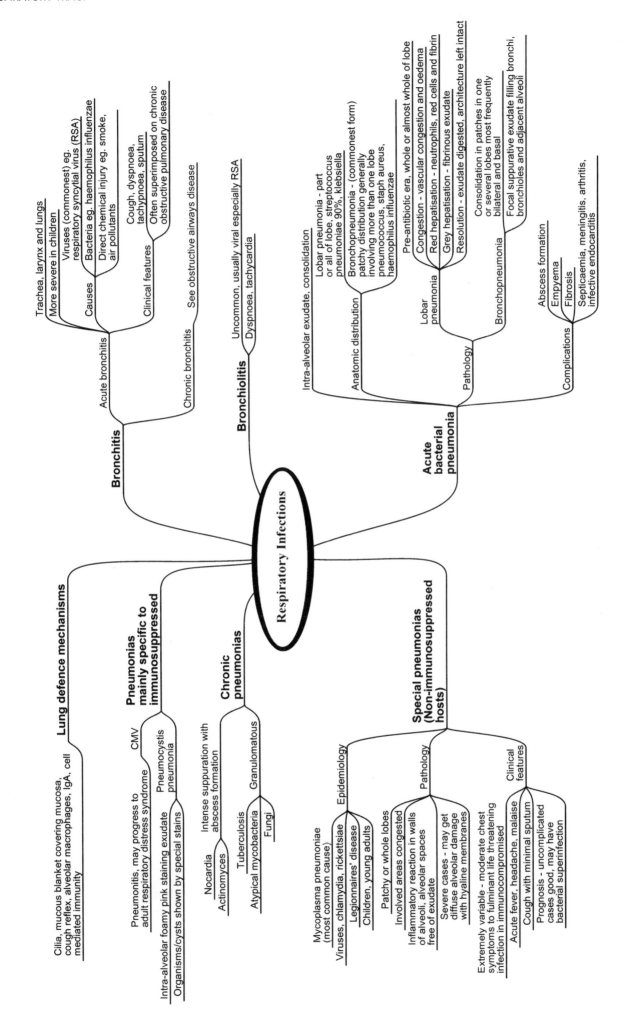

Respiratory Infections

Bronchitis

Acute bronchitis
- Trachea, larynx and lungs
- More severe in children
- Causes
  - Viruses (commonest) eg. respiratory syncytial virus (RSA)
  - Bacteria eg. haemophilus influenzae
  - Direct chemical injury eg. smoke, air pollutants
- Clinical features
  - Cough, dyspnoea, tachypnoea, sputum
  - Often superimposed on chronic obstructive pulmonary disease

Chronic bronchitis
- See obstructive airways disease

Bronchiolitis
- Uncommon, usually viral especially RSA
- Dyspnoea, tachycardia

Acute bacterial pneumonia

Intra-alveolar exudate, consolidation

Anatomic distribution
- Lobar pneumonia - part or all of lobe, streptococcus pneumoniae 90%, klebsiella
- Bronchopneumonia - (commonest form) patchy distribution generally involving more than one lobe pneumococcus, staph aureus, haemophilus influenzae

Pathology
- Lobar pneumonia
  - Pre-antibiotic era, whole or almost whole of lobe
  - Congestion - vascular congestion and oedema
  - Red hepatisation - neutrophils, red cells and fibrin
  - Grey hepatisation - fibrinous exudate
  - Resolution - exudate digested, architecture left intact
- Bronchopneumonia
  - Consolidation in patches in one or several lobes most frequently bilateral and basal
  - Focal suppurative exudate filling bronchi, bronchioles and adjacent alveoli

Complications
- Abscess formation
- Empyema
- Fibrosis
- Septicaemia, meningitis, arthritis, infective endocarditis

Lung defence mechanisms
- Cilia, mucous blanket covering mucosa, cough reflex, alveolar macrophages, IgA, cell mediated immunity

Pneumonias mainly specific to immunosuppressed
- CMV
  - Pneumonitis, may progress to adult respiratory distress syndrome
- Pneumocystis pneumonia
  - Intra-alveolar foamy pink staining exudate
  - Organisms/cysts shown by special stains

Chronic pneumonias
- Intense suppuration with abscess formation
  - Nocardia
  - Actinomyces
- Granulomatous
  - Tuberculosis
  - Atypical mycobacteria
  - Fungi

Special pneumonias (Non-immunosuppressed hosts)

Epidemiology
- Mycoplasma pneumoniae (most common cause)
- Viruses, chlamydia, rickettsiae
- Legionnaires' disease
- Children, young adults

Pathology
- Patchy or whole lobes
- Involved areas congested
- Inflammatory reaction in walls of alveoli, alveolar spaces free of exudate
- Severe cases - may get diffuse alveolar damage with hyaline membranes

Clinical features
- Extremely variable - moderate chest symptoms to fulminant life threatening infection in immunocompromised
- Acute fever, headache, malaise
- Cough with minimal sputum
- Prognosis - uncomplicated cases good, may have bacterial superinfection

SYSTEMATIC PATHOLOGY

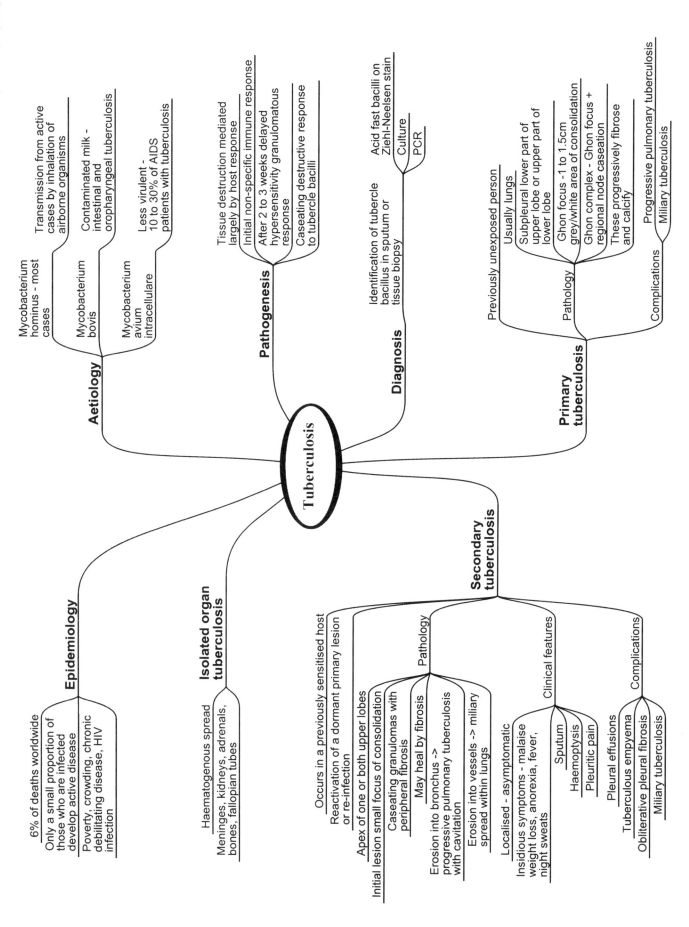

Tuberculosis

Aetiology

Mycobacterium hominus - most cases
- Transmission from active cases by inhalation of airborne organisms

Mycobacterium bovis
- Contaminated milk - intestinal and oropharyngeal tuberculosis

Mycobacterium avium intracellulare
- Less virulent - 10 to 30% of AIDS patients with tuberculosis

Pathogenesis
- Tissue destruction mediated largely by host response
- Initial non-specific immune response
- After 2 to 3 weeks delayed hypersensitivity granulomatous response
- Caseating destructive response to tubercle bacilli

Diagnosis
- Identification of tubercle bacillus in sputum or tissue biopsy
  - Acid fast bacilli on Ziehl-Neelsen stain
  - Culture
  - PCR

Primary tuberculosis
- Previously unexposed person
- Usually lungs
- Subpleural lower part of upper lobe or upper part of lower lobe
- **Pathology**
  - Ghon focus - 1 to 1.5cm grey/white area of consolidation
  - Ghon complex - Ghon focus + regional node caseation
  - These progressively fibrose and calcify
- **Complications**
  - Progressive pulmonary tuberculosis
  - Miliary tuberculosis

Epidemiology
- 6% of deaths worldwide
- Only a small proportion of those who are infected develop active disease
- Poverty, crowding, chronic debilitating disease, HIV infection

Isolated organ tuberculosis
- Haematogenous spread
- Meninges, kidneys, adrenals, bones, fallopian tubes

Secondary tuberculosis
- Occurs in a previously sensitised host
- Reactivation of a dormant primary lesion or re-infection
- Apex of one or both upper lobes
- Initial lesion small focus of consolidation
- **Pathology**
  - Caseating granulomas with peripheral fibrosis
  - May heal by fibrosis
  - Erosion into bronchus -> progressive pulmonary tuberculosis with cavitation
  - Erosion into vessels -> miliary spread within lungs
- **Clinical features**
  - Localised - asymptomatic
  - Insidious symptoms - malaise weight loss, anorexia, fever, night sweats
  - Sputum
  - Haemoptysis
  - Pleuritic pain
- **Complications**
  - Pleural effusions
  - Tuberculous empyema
  - Obliterative pleural fibrosis
  - Miliary tuberculosis

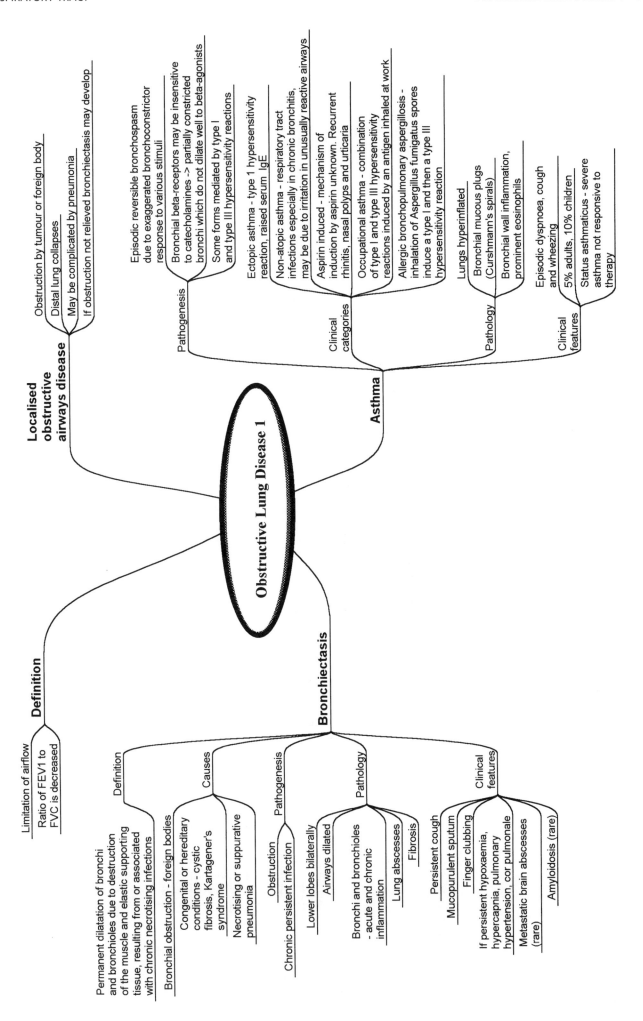

Obstructive Lung Disease 1

Definition
- Limitation of airflow
- Ratio of FEV1 to FVC is decreased

Localised obstructive airways disease
- Obstruction by tumour or foreign body
- Distal lung collapses
- May be complicated by pneumonia
- If obstruction not relieved bronchiectasis may develop

Asthma

Pathogenesis
- Episodic reversible bronchospasm due to exaggerated bronchoconstrictor response to various stimuli
- Bronchial beta-receptors may be insensitive to catecholamines -> partially constricted bronchi which do not dilate well to beta-agonists
- Some forms mediated by type I and type III hypersensitivity reactions

Clinical categories
- Ectopic asthma - type 1 hypersensitivity reaction, raised serum IgE
- Non-atopic asthma - respiratory tract infections especially in chronic bronchitis, may be due to irritation in unusually reactive airways
- Aspirin induced - mechanism of induction by aspirin unknown. Recurrent rhinitis, nasal polyps and urticaria
- Occupational asthma - combination of type I and type III hypersensitivity reactions induced by an antigen inhaled at work
- Allergic bronchopulmonary aspergillosis - inhalation of Aspergillus fumigatus spores induce a type I and then a type III hypersensitivity reaction

Pathology
- Lungs hyperinflated
- Bronchial mucous plugs (Curshmann's spirals)
- Bronchial wall inflammation, prominent eosinophils

Clinical features
- Episodic dyspnoea, cough and wheezing
- 5% adults, 10% children
- Status asthmaticus - severe asthma not responsive to therapy

Bronchiectasis

Definition
- Permanent dilatation of bronchi and bronchioles due to destruction of the muscle and elastic supporting tissue, resulting from or associated with chronic necrotising infections

Causes
- Bronchial obstruction - foreign bodies
- Congenital or hereditary conditions - cystic fibrosis, Kartagener's syndrome
- Necrotising or suppurative pneumonia

Pathogenesis
- Obstruction
- Chronic persistent infection

Pathology
- Lower lobes bilaterally
- Airways dilated
- Bronchi and bronchioles - acute and chronic inflammation
- Lung abscesses
- Fibrosis

Clinical features
- Persistent cough
- Mucopurulent sputum
- Finger clubbing
- If persistent hypoxaemia, hypercapnia, pulmonary hypertension, cor pulmonale
- Metastatic brain abscesses (rare)
- Amyloidosis (rare)

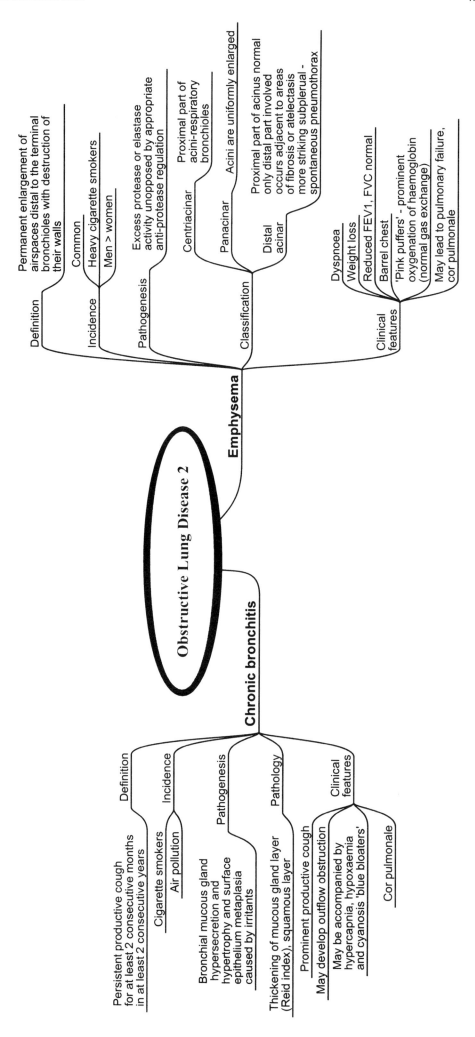

Obstructive Lung Disease 2

Emphysema

Definition — Permanent enlargement of airspaces distal to the terminal bronchioles with destruction of their walls

Incidence
- Common
- Heavy cigarette smokers
- Men > women

Pathogenesis — Excess protease or elastase activity unopposed by appropriate anti-protease regulation

Classification
- Centriacinar — Proximal part of acini-respiratory bronchioles
- Panacinar — Acini are uniformly enlarged
- Distal acinar — Proximal part of acinus normal only distal part involved occurs adjacent to areas of fibrosis or atelectasis more striking subplerual - spontaneous pneumothorax

Clinical features
- Dyspnoea
- Weight loss
- Reduced FEV1, FVC normal
- Barrel chest
- 'Pink puffers' - prominent oxygenation of haemoglobin (normal gas exchange)
- May lead to pulmonary failure, cor pulmonale

Chronic bronchitis

Definition — Persistent productive cough for at least 2 consecutive months in at least 2 consecutive years

Incidence
- Cigarette smokers
- Air pollution

Pathogenesis — Bronchial mucous gland hypersecretion and hypertrophy and surface epithelium metaplasia caused by irritants

Pathology — Thickening of mucous gland layer (Reid index), squamous layer

Clinical features
- Prominent productive cough
- May develop outflow obstruction
- May be accompanied by hypercapnia, hypoxaemia and cyanosis 'blue bloaters'
- Cor pulmonale

SYSTEMATIC PATHOLOGY

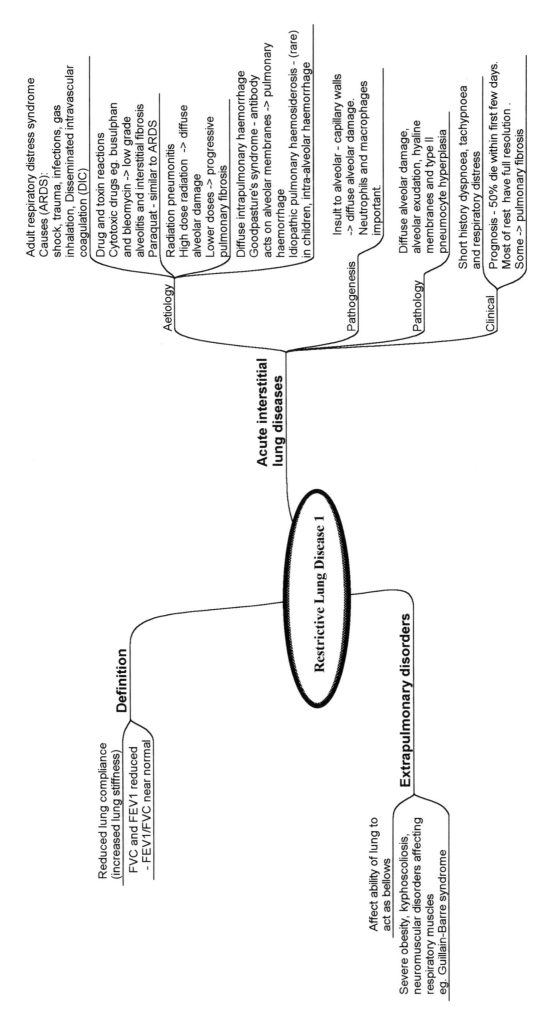

Restrictive Lung Disease 1

Acute interstitial lung diseases

Aetiology

Adult respiratory distress syndrome
Causes (ARDS):
shock, trauma, infections, gas inhalation, Disseminated intravascular coagulation (DIC)

Drug and toxin reactions
Cytotoxic drugs eg. busulphan and bleomycin -> low grade alveolitis and interstitial fibrosis
Paraquat - similar to ARDS

Radiation pneumonitis
High dose radiation -> diffuse alveolar damage
Lower doses -> progressive pulmonary fibrosis

Diffuse intrapulmonary haemorrhage
Goodpasture's syndrome - antibody acts on alveolar membranes -> pulmonary haemorrhage
Idiopathic pulmonary haemosiderosis - (rare) in children, intra-alveolar haemorrhage

Pathogenesis

Insult to alveolar - capillary walls -> diffuse alveolar damage.
Neutrophils and macrophages important.

Pathology

Diffuse alveolar damage, alveolar exudation, hyaline membranes and type II pneumocyte hyperplasia

Clinical

Short history dyspnoea, tachypnoea and respiratory distress

Prognosis - 50% die within first few days. Most of rest have full resolution . Some -> pulmonary fibrosis

Definition

Reduced lung compliance (increased lung stiffness)

FVC and FEV1 reduced - FEV1/FVC near normal

Extrapulmonary disorders

Affect ability of lung to act as bellows

Severe obesity, kyphoscoliosis, neuromuscular disorders affecting respiratory muscles
eg. Guillain-Barre syndrome

SYSTEMATIC PATHOLOGY

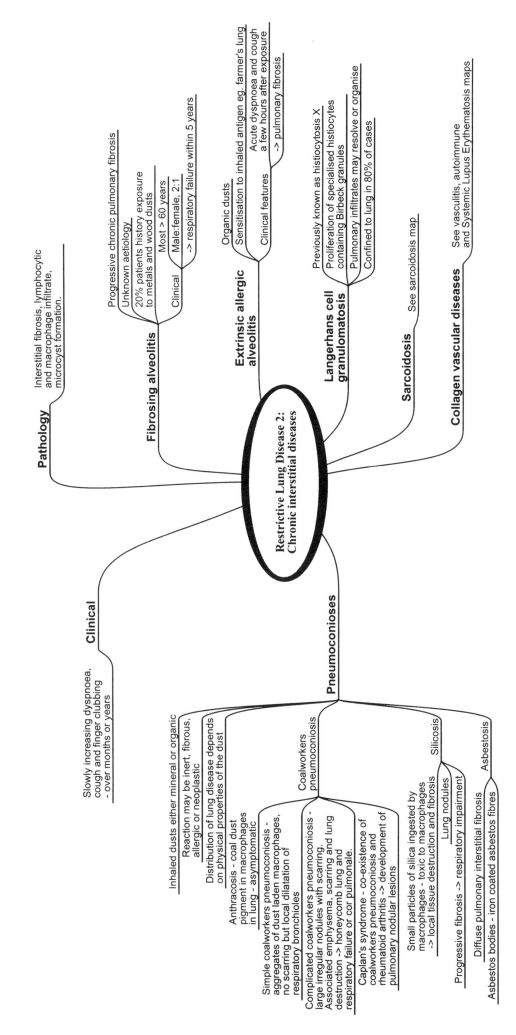

Restrictive Lung Disease 2: Chronic interstitial diseases

Pathology
- Interstitial fibrosis, lymphocytic and macrophage infiltrate, microcyst formation.

Fibrosing alveolitis
- Progressive chronic pulmonary fibrosis
- Unknown aetiology
- 20% patients history exposure to metals and wood dusts
- Clinical
  - Most > 60 years
  - Male:female, 2:1
  - -> respiratory failure within 5 years

Extrinsic allergic alveolitis
- Organic dusts
- Sensitisation to inhaled antigen eg. farmer's lung
- Clinical features
  - Acute dyspnoea and cough a few hours after exposure
  - -> pulmonary fibrosis

Langerhans cell granulomatosis
- Previously known as histiocytosis X
- Proliferation of specialised histiocytes containing Birbeck granules
- Pulmonary infiltrates may resolve or organise
- Confined to lung in 80% of cases

Sarcoidosis
- See sarcoidosis map

Collagen vascular diseases
- See vasculitis, autoimmune and Systemic Lupus Erythematosis maps

Clinical
- Slowly increasing dyspnoea, cough and finger clubbing - over months or years

Pneumoconioses
- Inhaled dusts either mineral or organic
- Reaction may be inert, fibrous, allergic or neoplastic
- Distribution of lung disease depends on physical properties of the dust
- Coalworkers pneumoconiosis
  - Anthracosis - coal dust pigment in macrophages in lung - asymptomatic
  - Simple coalworkers pneumoconiosis - aggregates of dust laden macrophages, no scarring but local dilatation of respiratory bronchioles
  - Complicated coalworkers pneumoconiosis - large irregular nodules with scarring. Associated emphysema, scarring and lung destruction -> honeycomb lung and respiratory failure or cor pulmonale.
  - Caplan's syndrome - co-existence of coalworkers pneumoconiosis and rheumatoid arthritis -> development of pulmonary nodular lesions
- Silicosis
  - Small particles of silica ingested by macrophages - toxic to macrophages -> local tissue destruction and fibrosis
  - Lung nodules
  - Progressive fibrosis -> respiratory impairment
- Asbestosis
  - Diffuse pulmonary interstitial fibrosis
  - Asbestos bodies - iron coated asbestos fibres

SYSTEMATIC PATHOLOGY

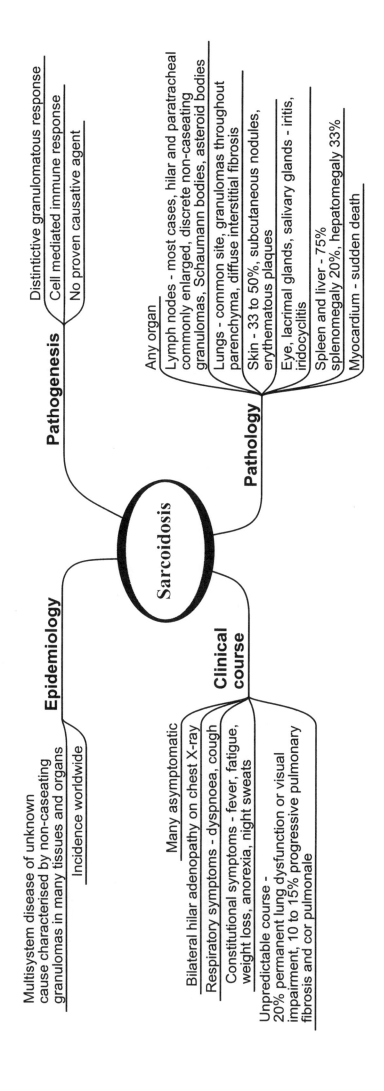

Sarcoidosis

Pathogenesis
- Distintictive granulomatous response
- Cell mediated immune response
- No proven causative agent

Pathology
- Any organ
- Lymph nodes - most cases, hilar and paratracheal commonly enlarged, discrete non-caseating granulomas, Schaumann bodies, asteroid bodies
- Lungs - common site, granulomas throughout parenchyma, diffuse interstitial fibrosis
- Skin - 33 to 50%, subcutaneous nodules, erythematous plaques
- Eye, lacrimal glands, salivary glands - iritis, iridocyclitis
- Spleen and liver - 75% splenomegaly 20%, hepatomegaly 33%
- Myocardium - sudden death

Epidemiology
- Multisystem disease of unknown cause characterised by non-caseating granulomas in many tissues and organs
- Incidence worldwide

Clinical course
- Many asymptomatic
- Bilateral hilar adenopathy on chest X-ray
- Respiratory symptoms - dyspnoea, cough
- Constitutional symptoms - fever, fatigue, weight loss, anorexia, night sweats
- Unpredictable course - 20% permanent lung dysfunction or visual impairment, 10 to 15% progressive pulmonary fibrosis and cor pulmonale

SYSTEMATIC PATHOLOGY

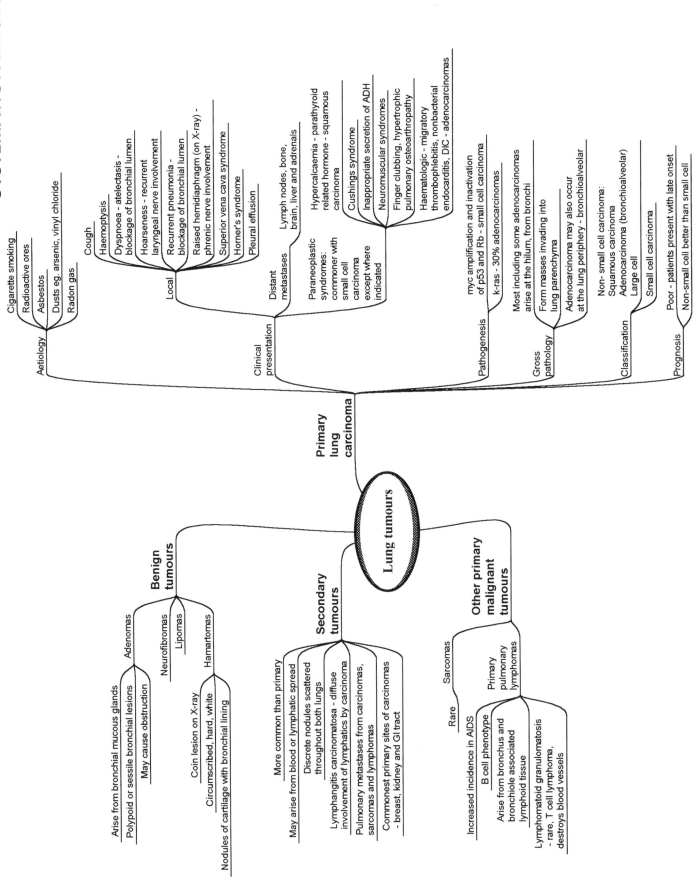

Lung tumours

Primary lung carcinoma

Aetiology
- Cigarette smoking
- Radioactive ores
- Asbestos
- Dusts eg. arsenic, vinyl chloride
- Radon gas

Clinical presentation
- Local
  - Cough
  - Haemoptysis
  - Dyspnoea - atelectasis - blockage of bronchial lumen
  - Hoarseness - recurrent laryngeal nerve involvement
  - Recurrent pneumonia - blockage of bronchial lumen
  - Raised hemidiaphragm (on X-ray) - phrenic nerve involvement
  - Superior vena cava syndrome
  - Horner's syndrome
  - Pleural effusion
- Distant metastases
  - Lymph nodes, bone, brain, liver and adrenals
- Paraneoplastic syndromes: commoner with small cell carcinoma except where indicated
  - Hypercalcaemia - parathyroid related hormone - squamous carcinoma
  - Cushings syndrome
  - Inappropriate secretion of ADH
  - Neuromuscular syndromes
  - Finger clubbing, hypertrophic pulmonary osteoarthropathy
  - Haematologic - migratory thrombophlebitis, nonbacterial endocarditis, DIC - adenocarcinomas

Pathogenesis
- myc amplification and inactivation of p53 and Rb - small cell carcinoma
- k-ras - 30% adenocarcinomas

Gross pathology
- Most including some adenocarcinomas arise at the hilum, from bronchi
- Form masses invading into lung parenchyma
- Adenocarcinoma may also occur at the lung periphery - bronchioalveolar

Classification
- Non-small cell carcinoma:
  - Squamous carcinoma
  - Adenocarcinoma (bronchioalveolar)
  - Large cell
- Small cell carcinoma

Prognosis
- Poor - patients present with late onset
- Non-small cell better than small cell

Benign tumours

- Adenomas
  - Arise from bronchial mucous glands
  - Polypoid or sessile bronchial lesions
  - May cause obstruction
- Neurofibromas
- Lipomas
- Hamartomas
  - Coin lesion on X-ray
  - Circumscribed, hard, white
  - Nodules of cartilage with bronchial lining

Secondary tumours

- More common than primary
- May arise from blood or lymphatic spread
- Discrete nodules scattered throughout both lungs
- Lymphangitis carcinomatosa - diffuse involvement of lymphatics by carcinoma
- Pulmonary metastases from carcinomas, sarcomas and lymphomas
- Commonest primary sites of carcinomas - breast, kidney and GI tract

Other primary malignant tumours

- Sarcomas
  - Rare
- Primary pulmonary lymphomas
  - Increased incidence in AIDS
  - B cell phenotype
  - Arise from bronchus and bronchiole associated lymphoid tissue
  - Lymphomatoid granulomatosis - rare, T cell lymphoma, destroys blood vessels

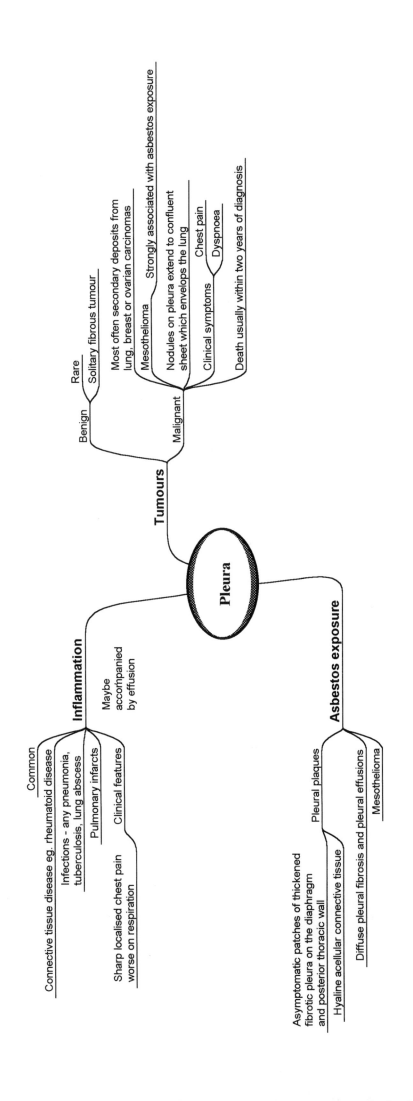

Pleura

Tumours

Benign

Rare

Solitary fibrous tumour

Malignant

Most often secondary deposits from lung, breast or ovarian carcinomas

Mesothelioma

Strongly associated with asbestos exposure

Nodules on pleura extend to confluent sheet which envelops the lung

Clinical symptoms

Chest pain

Dyspnoea

Death usually within two years of diagnosis

Inflammation

Common

Connective tissue disease eg. rheumatoid disease

Infections - any pneumonia, tuberculosis, lung abscess

Pulmonary infarcts

Clinical features

Sharp localised chest pain worse on respiration

Maybe accompanied by effusion

Asbestos exposure

Pleural plaques

Asymptomatic patches of thickened fibrotic pleura on the diaphragm and posterior thoracic wall

Hyaline acellular connective tissue

Diffuse pleural fibrosis and pleural effusions

Mesothelioma

GASTRO-INTESTINAL TRACT

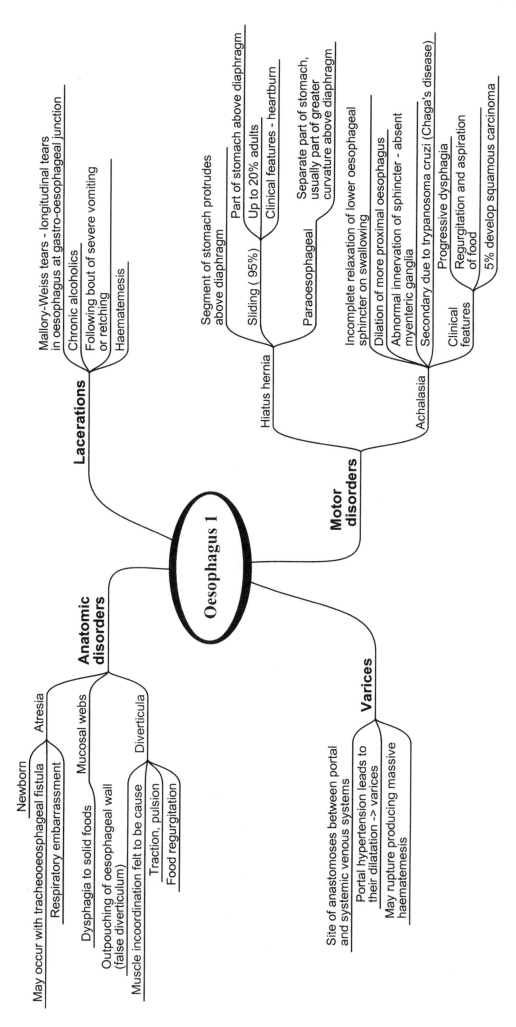

Oesophagus 1

Lacerations

Mallory-Weiss tears - longitudinal tears
in oesophagus at gastro-oesophageal junction

Chronic alcoholics

Following bout of severe vomiting
or retching

Haematemesis

Anatomic disorders

Atresia

Newborn

May occur with tracheoeoesophageal fistula

Respiratory embarrassment

Mucosal webs

Dysphagia to solid foods

Diverticula

Outpouching of oesophageal wall
(false diverticulum)

Muscle incoordination felt to be cause

Traction, pulsion

Food regurgitation

Varices

Site of anastomoses between portal
and systemic venous systems

Portal hypertension leads to
their dilatation -> varices

May rupture producing massive
haematemesis

Motor disorders

Hiatus hernia

Segment of stomach protrudes
above diaphragm

Sliding (95%)

Part of stomach above diaphragm

Up to 20% adults

Clinical features - heartburn

Paraoesophageal

Separate part of stomach,
usually part of greater
curvature above diaphragm

Achalasia

Incomplete relaxation of lower oesophageal
sphincter on swallowing

Dilation of more proximal oesophagus

Abnormal innervation of sphincter - absent
myenteric ganglia

Secondary due to trypanosoma cruzi (Chaga's disease)

Clinical features

Progressive dysphagia

Regurgitation and aspiration
of food

5% develop squamous carcinoma

SYSTEMATIC PATHOLOGY

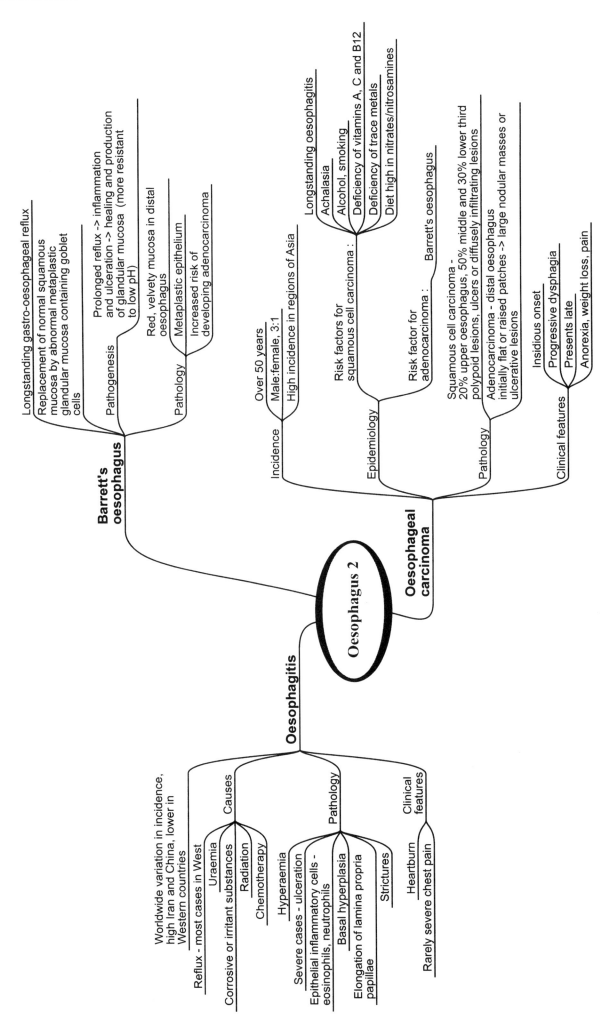

Oesophagus 2

Barrett's oesophagus

Pathogenesis
- Longstanding gastro-oesophageal reflux
- Replacement of normal squamous mucosa by abnormal metaplastic glandular mucosa containing goblet cells
- Prolonged reflux -> inflammation and ulceration -> healing and production of glandular mucosa (more resistant to low pH)

Pathology
- Red, velvety mucosa in distal oesophagus
- Metaplastic epithelium
- Increased risk of developing adenocarcinoma

Oesophageal carcinoma

Epidemiology
- Incidence
  - Over 50 years
  - Male:female, 3:1
  - High incidence in regions of Asia
- Risk factors for squamous cell carcinoma :
  - Longstanding oesophagitis
  - Achalasia
  - Alcohol, smoking
  - Deficiency of vitamins A, C and B12
  - Deficiency of trace metals
  - Diet high in nitrates/nitrosamines
- Risk factor for adenocarcinoma :
  - Barrett's oesophagus

Pathology
- Squamous cell carcinoma - 20% upper oesophagus, 50% middle and 30% lower third polypoid lesions, ulcers or diffusely infiltrating lesions
- Adenocarcinoma - distal oesophagus initially flat or raised patches -> large nodular masses or ulcerative lesions

Clinical features
- Insidious onset
- Progressive dysphagia
- Presents late
- Anorexia, weight loss, pain

Oesophagitis

Causes
- Worldwide variation in incidence, high Iran and China, lower in Western countries
- Reflux - most cases in West
- Uraemia
- Corrosive or irritant substances
- Radiation
- Chemotherapy

Pathology
- Hyperaemia
- Severe cases - ulceration
- Epithelial inflammatory cells - eosinophils, neutrophils
- Basal hyperplasia
- Elongation of lamina propria papillae
- Strictures

Clinical features
- Heartburn
- Rarely severe chest pain

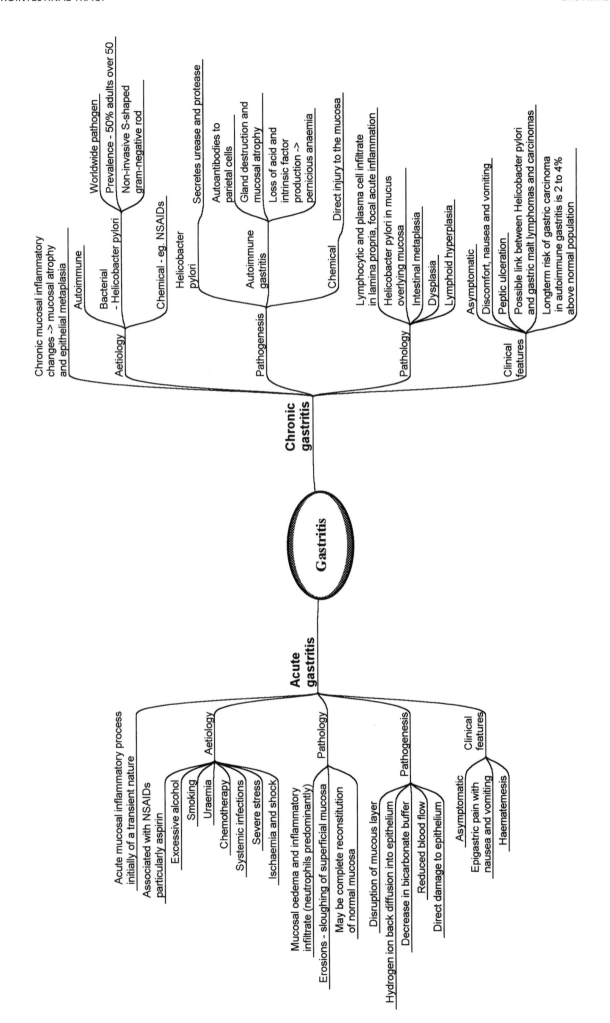

Gastritis

Chronic gastritis

Aetiology
- Chronic mucosal inflammatory changes -> mucosal atrophy and epithelial metaplasia
- Autoimmune
- Bacterial - Helicobacter pylori
  - Worldwide pathogen
  - Prevalence - 50% adults over 50
  - Non-invasive S-shaped gram-negative rod
- Chemical - eg. NSAIDs

Pathogenesis
- Helicobacter pylori
  - Secretes urease and protease
- Autoimmune gastritis
  - Autoantibodies to parietal cells
  - Gland destruction and mucosal atrophy
  - Loss of acid and intrinsic factor production -> pernicious anaemia
- Chemical
  - Direct injury to the mucosa

Pathology
- Lymphocytic and plasma cell infiltrate in lamina propria, focal acute inflammation
- Helicobacter pylori in mucus overlying mucosa
- Intestinal metaplasia
- Dysplasia
- Lymphoid hyperplasia

Clinical features
- Asymptomatic
- Discomfort, nausea and vomiting
- Peptic ulceration
- Possible link between Helicobacter pylori and gastric malt lymphomas and carcinomas
- Longterm risk of gastric carcinoma in autoimmune gastritis is 2 to 4% above normal population

Acute gastritis

Aetiology
- Acute mucosal inflammatory process initially of a transient nature
- Associated with NSAIDs particularly aspirin
- Excessive alcohol
- Smoking
- Uraemia
- Chemotherapy
- Systemic infections
- Severe stress
- Ischaemia and shock

Pathology
- Mucosal oedema and inflammatory infiltrate (neutrophils predominantly)
- Erosions - sloughing of superficial mucosa
- May be complete reconstitution of normal mucosa

Pathogenesis
- Disruption of mucous layer
- Hydrogen ion back diffusion into epithelium
- Decrease in bicarbonate buffer
- Reduced blood flow
- Direct damage to epithelium

Clinical features
- Asymptomatic
- Epigastric pain with nausea and vomiting
- Haematemesis

SYSTEMATIC PATHOLOGY

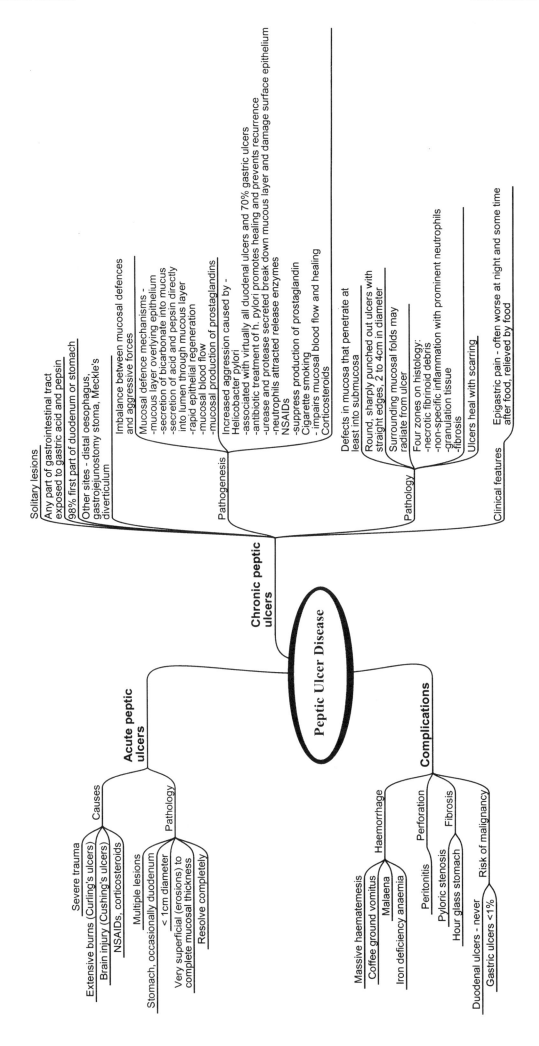

Peptic Ulcer Disease

Chronic peptic ulcers

Solitary lesions

Any part of gastrointestinal tract exposed to gastric acid and pepsin

98% first part of duodenum or stomach

Other sites - distal oesophagus, gastrojejunostomy stoma, Meckle's diverticulum

Pathogenesis

Imbalance between mucosal defences and aggressive forces

Mucosal defence mechanisms -
-mucous layer overlying epithelium
-secretion of bicarbonate into mucus
-secretion of acid and pepsin directly into lumen through mucous layer
-rapid epithelial regeneration
-mucosal blood flow
-mucosal production of prostaglandins

Increased aggression caused by -
Helicobacter pylori
-associated with virtually all duodenal ulcers and 70% gastric ulcers
-antibiotic treatment of h. pylori promotes healing and prevents recurrence
-urease and protease secreted break down mucous layer and damage surface epithelium
-neutrophils attracted release enzymes
NSAIDs
-suppress production of prostaglandin
Cigarette smoking
-impairs mucosal blood flow and healing
Corticosteroids

Pathology

Defects in mucosa that penetrate at least into submucosa

Round, sharply punched out ulcers with straight edges, 2 to 4cm in diameter

Surrounding mucosal folds may radiate from ulcer

Four zones on histology:
-necrotic fibrinoid debris
-non-specific inflammation with prominent neutrophils
-granulation tissue
-fibrosis

Ulcers heal with scarring

Clinical features

Epigastric pain - often worse at night and some time after food, relieved by food

Acute peptic ulcers

Causes

Severe trauma

Extensive burns (Curling's ulcers)

Brain injury (Cushing's ulcers)

NSAIDs, corticosteroids

Pathology

Multiple lesions

Stomach, occasionally duodenum

< 1cm diameter

Very superficial (erosions) to complete mucosal thickness

Resolve completely

Complications

Haemorrhage

Massive haematemesis

Coffee ground vomitus

Malaena

Iron deficiency anaemia

Perforation

Peritonitis

Fibrosis

Pyloric stenosis

Hour glass stomach

Risk of malignancy

Duodenal ulcers - never

Gastric ulcers <1%

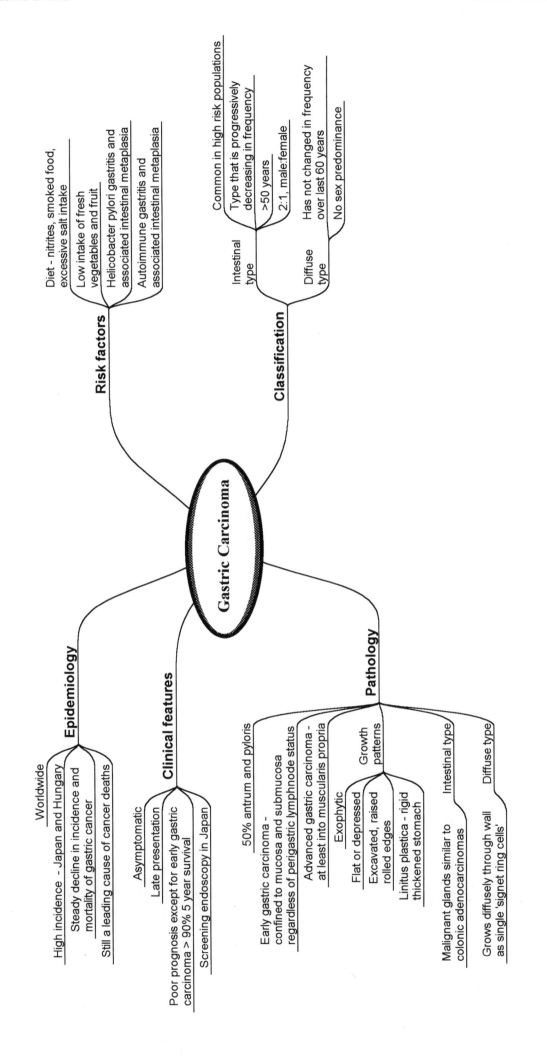

Gastric Carcinoma

Risk factors
- Diet - nitrites, smoked food, excessive salt intake
- Low intake of fresh vegetables and fruit
- Helicobacter pylori gastritis and associated intestinal metaplasia
- Autoimmune gastritis and associated intestinal metaplasia

Classification
- Intestinal type
  - Common in high risk populations
  - Type that is progressively decreasing in frequency
  - >50 years
  - 2:1, male:female
- Diffuse type
  - Has not changed in frequency over last 60 years
  - No sex predominance

Epidemiology
- Worldwide
- High incidence - Japan and Hungary
- Steady decline in incidence and mortality of gastric cancer
- Still a leading cause of cancer deaths

Clinical features
- Asymptomatic
- Late presentation
- Poor prognosis except for early gastric carcinoma > 90% 5 year survival
- Screening endoscopy in Japan

Pathology
- 50% antrum and pyloris
- Early gastric carcinoma - confined to mucosa and submucosa regardless of perigastric lymphnode status
- Advanced gastric carcinoma - at least into muscularis propria
- Growth patterns
  - Exophytic
  - Flat or depressed
  - Excavated, raised rolled edges
  - Linitus plastica - rigid thickened stomach
- Intestinal type
  - Malignant glands similar to colonic adenocarcinomas
- Diffuse type
  - Grows diffusely through wall as single 'signet ring cells'

SYSTEMATIC PATHOLOGY

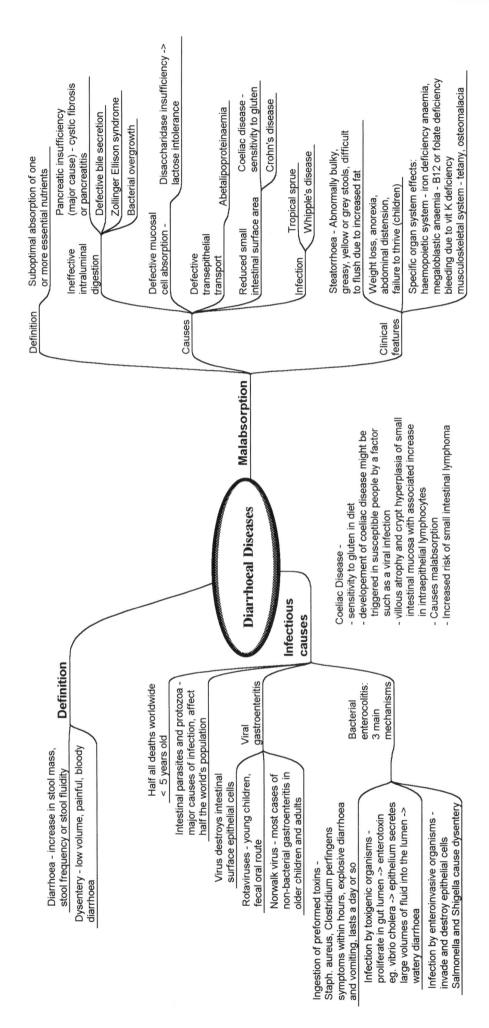

Diarrhoeal Diseases

Definition

Diarrhoea - increase in stool mass, stool frequency or stool fluidity

Dysentery - low volume, painful, bloody diarrhoea

Infectious causes

Half all deaths worldwide < 5 years old

Intestinal parasites and protozoa - major causes of infection, affect half the world's population

Viral gastroenteritis

Virus destroys intestinal surface epithelial cells

Rotaviruses - young children, fecal oral route

Norwalk virus - most cases of non-bacterial gastroenteritis in older children and adults

Bacterial enterocolitis: 3 main mechanisms

Ingestion of preformed toxins - Staph. aureus, Clostridium perfingens symptoms within hours, explosive diarrhoea and vomiting, lasts a day or so

Infection by toxigenic organisms - proliferate in gut lumen -> enterotoxin eg. vibrio cholera -> epithelium secretes large volumes of fluid into the lumen -> watery diarrhoea

Infection by enteroinvasive organisms - invade and destroy epithelial cells Salmonella and Shigella cause dysentery

Coeliac Disease -
- sensitivity to gluten in diet
- development of coeliac disease might be triggered in susceptible people by a factor such as a viral infection
- villous atrophy and crypt hyperplasia of small intestinal mucosa with associated increase in intraepithelial lymphocytes
- Causes malabsorption
- Increased risk of small intestinal lymphoma

Malabsorption

Definition

Suboptimal absorption of one or more essential nutrients

Causes

Ineffective intraluminal digestion

Pancreatic insufficiency (major cause) - cystic fibrosis or pancreatitis

Defective bile secretion

Zollinger Ellison syndrome

Bacterial overgrowth

Defective mucosal cell absorption -

Disaccharidase insufficiency -> lactose intolerance

Defective transepithelial transport

Abetalipoproteinaemia

Reduced small intestinal surface area

Coeliac disease - sensitivity to gluten

Crohn's disease

Infection

Tropical sprue

Whipple's disease

Clinical features

Steatorrhoea - Abnormally bulky, greasy, yellow or grey stools, difficult to flush due to increased fat

Weight loss, anorexia, abdominal distension, failure to thrive (children)

Specific organ system effects:
haemopoietic system - iron deficiency anaemia, megaloblastic anaemia - B12 or folate deficiency bleeding due to vit K deficiency
musculoskeletal system - tetany, osteomalacia

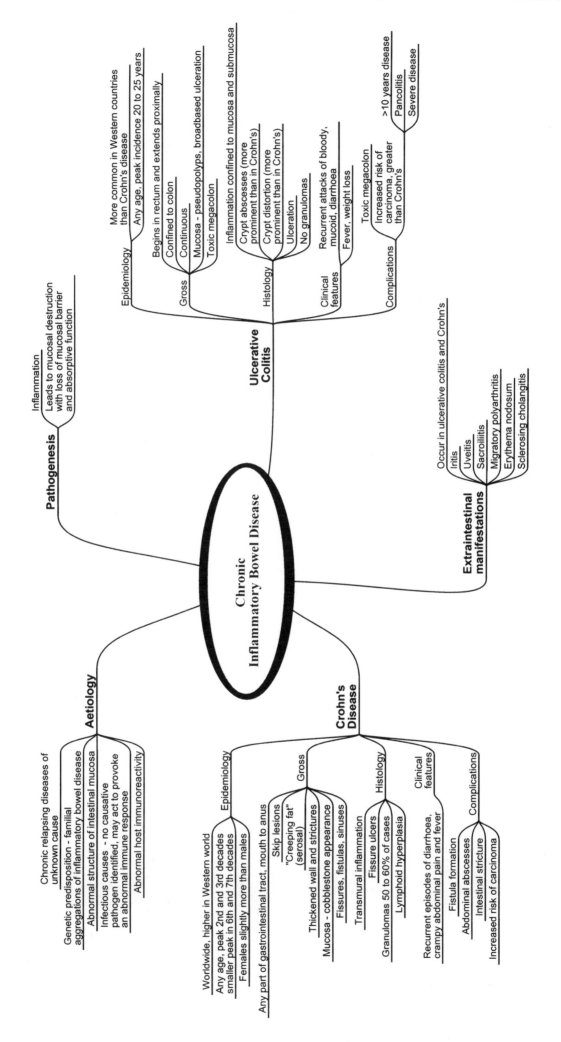

Chronic Inflammatory Bowel Disease

Pathogenesis
- Inflammation
- Leads to mucosal destruction with loss of mucosal barrier and absorptive function

Ulcerative Colitis

Epidemiology
- More common in Western countries than Crohn's disease
- Any age, peak incidence 20 to 25 years

Gross
- Begins in rectum and extends proximally
- Confined to colon
- Continuous
- Mucosa – pseudopolyps, broadbased ulceration
- Toxic megacolon

Histology
- Inflammation confined to mucosa and submucosa
- Crypt abscesses (more prominent than in Crohn's)
- Crypt distortion (more prominent than in Crohn's)
- Ulceration
- No granulomas

Clinical features
- Recurrent attacks of bloody, mucoid, diarrhoea
- Fever, weight loss

Complications
- Toxic megacolon
- Increased risk of carcinoma, greater than Crohn's
  - >10 years disease
  - Pancolitis
  - Severe disease

Extraintestinal manifestations
- Occur in ulcerative colitis and Crohn's
- Iritis
- Uveitis
- Sacroiliitis
- Migratory polyarthritis
- Erythema nodosum
- Sclerosing cholangitis

Aetiology
- Chronic relapsing diseases of unknown cause
- Genetic predisposition - familial aggregations of inflammatory bowel disease
- Abnormal structure of intestinal mucosa
- Infectious causes - no causative pathogen identified, may act to provoke an abnormal immune response
- Abnormal host immunoreactivity

Crohn's Disease

Epidemiology
- Worldwide, higher in Western world
- Any age, peak 2nd and 3rd decades smaller peak in 6th and 7th decades
- Females slightly more than males

Gross
- Any part of gastrointestinal tract, mouth to anus
- Skip lesions
- "Creeping fat" (serosal)
- Thickened wall and strictures
- Mucosa - cobblestone appearance
- Fissures, fistulas, sinuses

Histology
- Transmural inflammation
- Fissure ulcers
- Granulomas 50 to 60% of cases
- Lymphoid hyperplasia

Clinical features
- Recurrent episodes of diarrhoea, crampy abdominal pain and fever

Complications
- Fistula formation
- Abdominal abscesses
- Intestinal stricture
- Increased risk of carcinoma

SYSTEMATIC PATHOLOGY

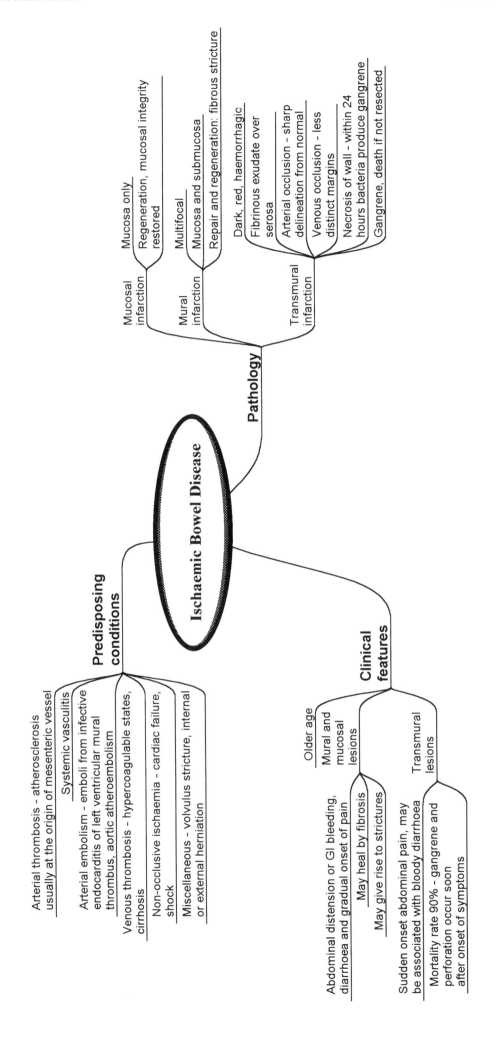

Ischaemic Bowel Disease

Pathology

Mucosal infarction
- Mucosa only
- Regeneration, mucosal integrity restored

Mural infarction
- Multifocal
- Mucosa and submucosa
- Repair and regeneration: fibrous stricture

Transmural infarction
- Dark, red, haemorrhagic
- Fibrinous exudate over serosa
- Arterial occlusion - sharp delineation from normal
- Venous occlusion - less distinct margins
- Necrosis of wall - within 24 hours bacteria produce gangrene
- Gangrene, death if not resected

Predisposing conditions
- Arterial thrombosis - atherosclerosis usually at the origin of mesenteric vessel
- Systemic vasculitis
- Arterial embolism - emboli from infective endocarditis of left ventricular mural thrombus, aortic atheroembolism
- Venous thrombosis - hypercoagulable states, cirrhosis
- Non-occlusive ischaemia - cardiac failure, shock
- Miscellaneous - volvulus stricture, internal or external herniation

Clinical features
- Older age

Mural and mucosal lesions
- Abdominal distension or GI bleeding, diarrhoea and gradual onset of pain
- May heal by fibrosis
- May give rise to strictures

Transmural lesions
- Sudden onset abdominal pain, may be associated with bloody diarrhoea
- Mortality rate 90% - gangrene and perforation occur soon after onset of symptoms

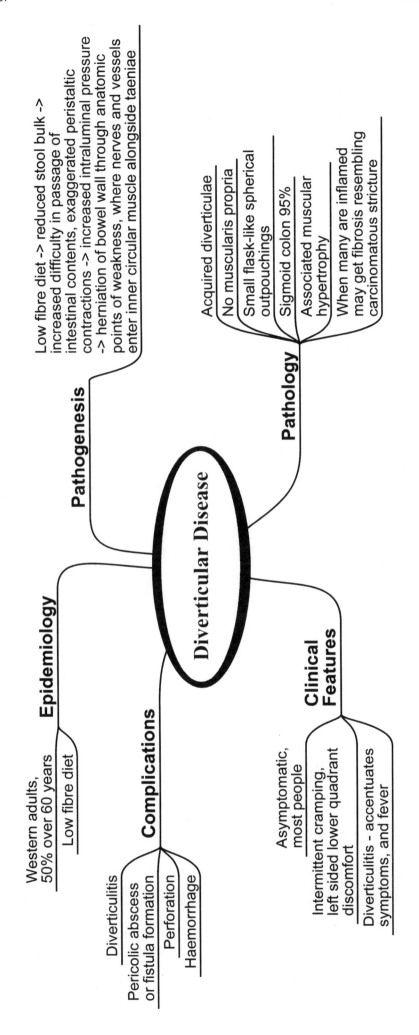

Diverticular Disease

Pathogenesis

Low fibre diet -> reduced stool bulk -> increased difficulty in passage of intestinal contents, exaggerated peristaltic contractions -> increased intraluminal pressure -> herniation of bowel wall through anatomic points of weakness, where nerves and vessels enter inner circular muscle alongside taeniae

Pathology

Acquired diverticulae

No muscularis propria

Small flask-like spherical outpouchings

Sigmoid colon 95%

Associated muscular hypertrophy

When many are inflamed may get fibrosis resembling carcinomatous stricture

Epidemiology

Western adults, 50% over 60 years

Low fibre diet

Complications

Diverticulitis

Pericolic abscess or fistula formation

Perforation

Haemorrhage

Clinical Features

Asymptomatic, most people

Intermittent cramping, left sided lower quadrant discomfort

Diverticulitis - accentuates symptoms, and fever

SYSTEMATIC PATHOLOGY

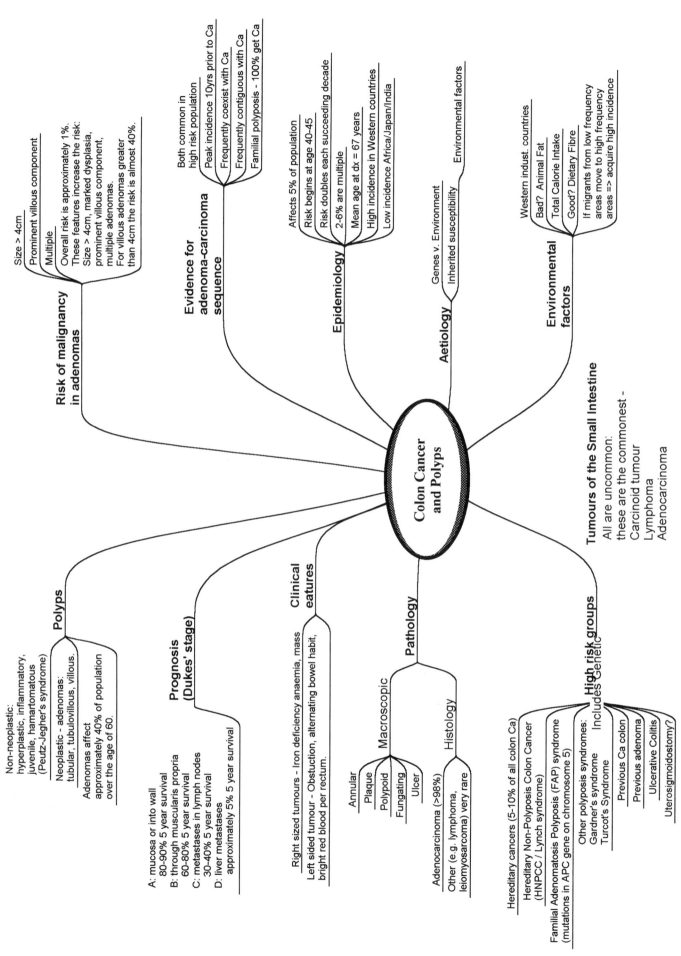

Risk of malignancy in adenomas
- Size > 4cm
- Prominent villous component
- Multiple
- Overall risk is approximately 1%. These features increase the risk: Size > 4cm, marked dysplasia, prominent villous component, multiple adenomas. For villous adenomas greater than 4cm the risk is almost 40%.

Evidence for adenoma-carcinoma sequence
- Both common in high risk population
- Peak incidence 10yrs prior to Ca
- Frequently coexist with Ca
- Frequently contiguous with Ca
- Familial polyposis - 100% get Ca

Epidemiology
- Affects 5% of population
- Risk begins at age 40-45
- Risk doubles each succeeding decade
- 2-6% are multiple
- Mean age at dx = 67 years
- High incidence in Western countries
- Low incidence Africa/Japan/India

Aetiology
- Genes v. Environment
- Inherited susceptibility
- Environmental factors

Environmental factors
- Western indust. countries
- Bad? Animal Fat
- Total Calorie Intake
- Good? Dietary Fibre
- If migrants from low frequency areas move to high frequency areas => acquire high incidence

Colon Cancer and Polyps

Tumours of the Small Intestine
All are uncommon: these are the commonest -
Carcinoid tumour
Lymphoma
Adenocarcinoma

Polyps
- Non-neoplastic: hyperplastic, inflammatory, juvenile, hamartomatous (Peutz-Jegher's syndrome)
- Neoplastic - adenomas: tubular, tubulovillous, villous. Adenomas affect approximately 40% of population over the age of 60.

Prognosis (Dukes' stage)
- A: mucosa or into wall 80-90% 5 year survival
- B: through muscularis propria 60-80% 5 year survival
- C: metastases in lymph nodes 30-40% 5 year survival
- D: liver metastases approximately 5% 5 year survival

Clinical features
- Right sized tumours - Iron deficiency anaemia, mass
- Left sided tumour - Obstuction, alternating bowel habit, bright red blood per rectum.

Pathology

Macroscopic
- Annular
- Plaque
- Polypoid
- Fungating
- Ulcer

Histology
- Adenocarcinoma (>98%)
- Other (e.g. lymphoma, leiomyosarcoma) very rare

High risk groups

Genetic
- Hereditary cancers (5-10% of all colon Ca)
- Hereditary Non-Polyposis Colon Cancer (HNPCC / Lynch syndrome)
- Familial Adenomatosis Polyposis (FAP) syndrome (mutations in APC gene on chromosome 5)
- Other polyposis syndromes: *Includes* Gardner's syndrome Turcot's Syndrome

- Previous Ca colon
- Previous adenoma
- Ulcerative Colitis
- Uterosigmoidostomy?

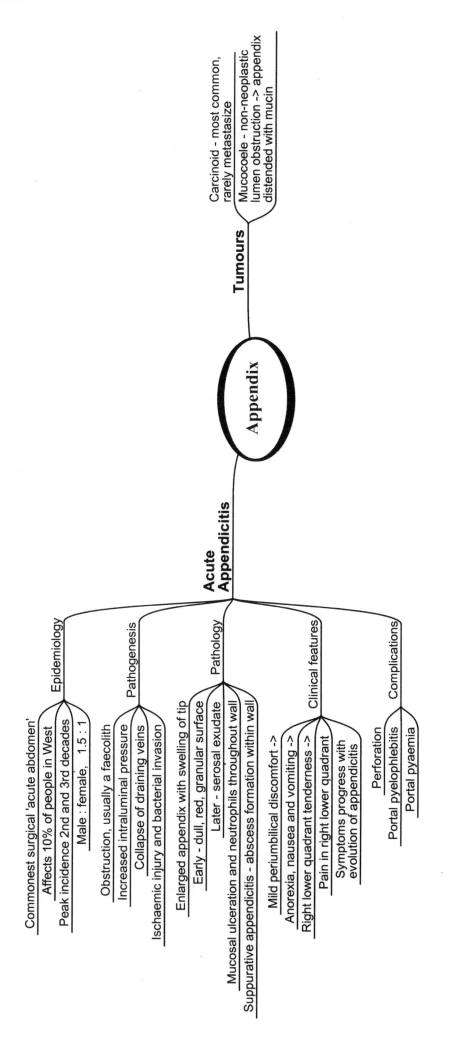

Appendix

Tumours

Carcinoid - most common, rarely metastasize

Mucocoele - non-neoplastic lumen obstruction -> appendix distended with mucin

Acute Appendicitis

Epidemiology
- Commonest surgical 'acute abdomen'
- Affects 10% of people in West
- Peak incidence 2nd and 3rd decades
- Male : female, 1.5 : 1

Pathogenesis
- Obstruction, usually a faecolith
- Increased intraluminal pressure
- Collapse of draining veins
- Ischaemic injury and bacterial invasion

Pathology
- Enlarged appendix with swelling of tip
- Early - dull, red, granular surface
- Later - serosal exudate
- Mucosal ulceration and neutrophils throughout wall
- Suppurative appendicitis - abscess formation within wall

Clinical features
- Mild periumbilical discomfort ->
- Anorexia, nausea and vomiting ->
- Right lower quadrant tenderness ->
- Pain in right lower quadrant
- Symptoms progress with evolution of appendicitis

Complications
- Perforation
- Portal pyelophlebitis
- Portal pyaemia

LIVER, BILIARY TRACT AND EXOCRINE PANCREAS

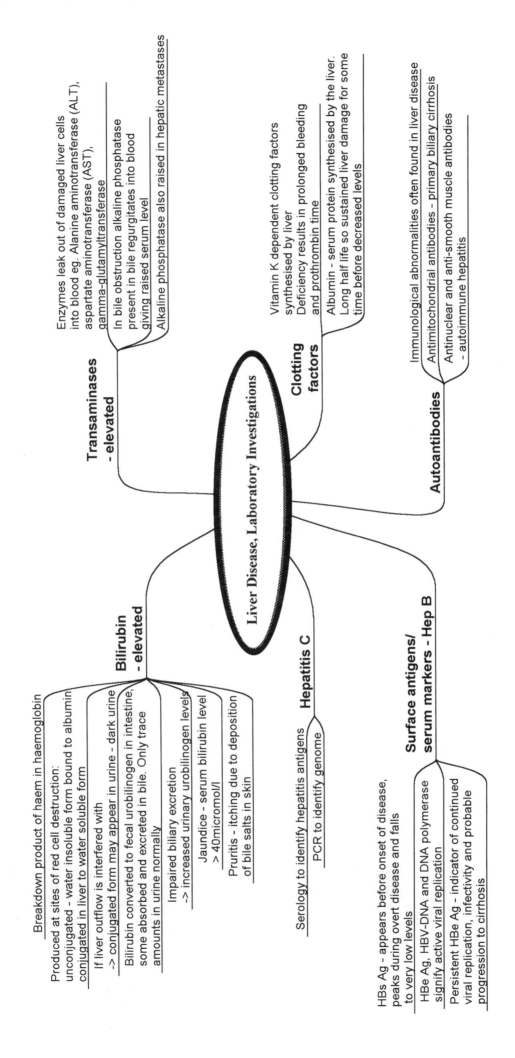

Liver Disease, Laboratory Investigations

Transaminases - elevated

Enzymes leak out of damaged liver cells into blood eg. Alanine aminotransferase (ALT), aspartate aminotransferase (AST), gamma-glutamyltransferase

In bile obstruction alkaline phosphatase present in bile regurgitates into blood giving raised serum level

Alkaline phosphatase also raised in hepatic metastases

Clotting factors

Vitamin K dependent clotting factors synthesised by liver
Deficiency results in prolonged bleeding and prothrombin time

Albumin - serum protein synthesised by the liver. Long half life so sustained liver damage for some time before decreased levels

Autoantibodies

Immunological abnormalities often found in liver disease
Antimitochondrial antibodies - primary biliary cirrhosis
Antinuclear and anti-smooth muscle antibodies - autoimmune hepatitis

Bilirubin - elevated

Breakdown product of haem in haemoglobin

Produced at sites of red cell destruction: unconjugated - water insoluble form bound to albumin conjugated in liver to water soluble form

If liver outflow is interfered with -> conjugated form may appear in urine - dark urine

Bilirubin converted to fecal urobilinogen in intestine, some absorbed and excreted in bile. Only trace amounts in urine normally

Impaired biliary excretion -> increased urinary urobilinogen levels

Jaundice - serum bilirubin level >40micromol/l

Pruritis - itching due to deposition of bile salts in skin

Hepatitis C

Serology to identify hepatitis antigens
PCR to identify genome

Surface antigens/ serum markers - Hep B

HBs Ag - appears before onset of disease, peaks during overt disease and falls to very low levels

HBe Ag, HBV-DNA and DNA polymerase signify active viral replication

Persistent HBe Ag - indicator of continued viral replication, infectivity and probable progression to cirrhosis

SYSTEMATIC PATHOLOGY

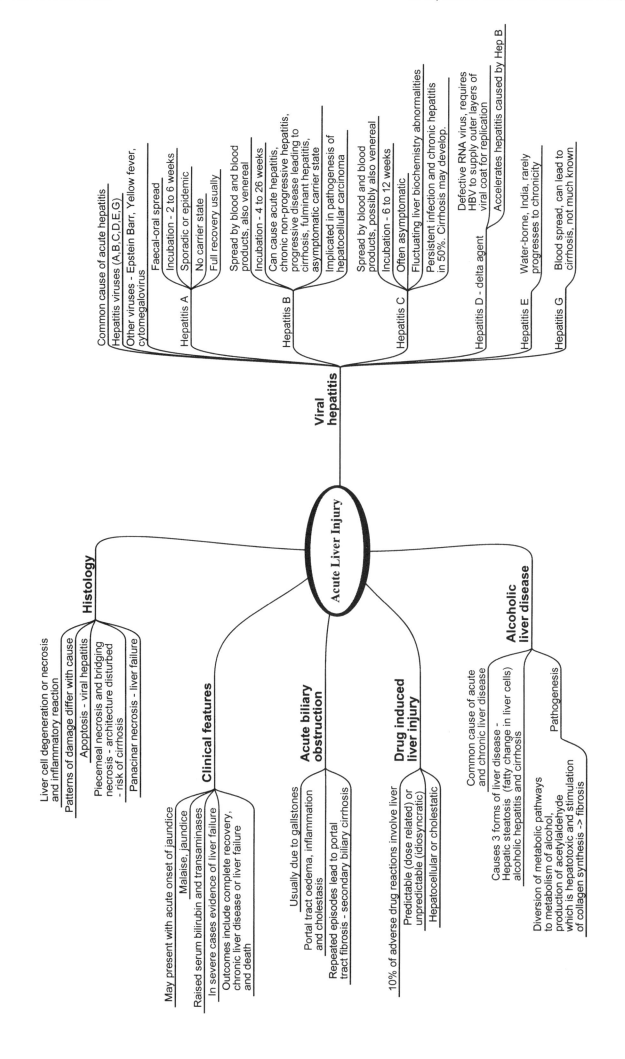

Acute Liver Injury

Viral hepatitis

Common cause of acute hepatitis

Hepatitis viruses (A,B,C,D,E,G)

Other viruses - Epstein Barr, Yellow fever, cytomegalovirus

Hepatitis A
- Faecal-oral spread
- Incubation - 2 to 6 weeks
- Sporadic or epidemic
- No carrier state
- Full recovery usually

Hepatitis B
- Spread by blood and blood products, also venereal
- Incubation - 4 to 26 weeks
- Can cause acute hepatitis, chronic non-progressive hepatitis, progressive disease leading to cirrhosis, fulminant hepatitis, asymptomatic carrier state
- Implicated in pathogenesis of hepatocellular carcinoma

Hepatitis C
- Spread by blood and blood products, possibly also venereal
- Incubation - 6 to 12 weeks
- Often asymptomatic
- Fluctuating liver biochemistry abnormalities
- Persistent infection and chronic hepatitis in 50%. Cirrhosis may develop.

Hepatitis D - delta agent
- Defective RNA virus, requires HBV to supply outer layers of viral coat for replication
- Accelerates hepatitis caused by Hep B

Hepatitis E
- Water-borne, India, rarely progresses to chronicity

Hepatitis G
- Blood spread, can lead to cirrhosis, not much known

Histology
- Liver cell degeneration or necrosis and inflammatory reaction
- Patterns of damage differ with cause
- Apoptosis - viral hepatitis
- Piecemeal necrosis and bridging necrosis - architecture disturbed - risk of cirrhosis
- Panacinar necrosis - liver failure

Clinical features
- May present with acute onset of jaundice
- Malaise, jaundice
- Raised serum bilirubin and transaminases
- In severe cases evidence of liver failure
- Outcomes include complete recovery, chronic liver disease or liver failure and death

Acute biliary obstruction
- Usually due to gallstones
- Portal tract oedema, inflammation and cholestasis
- Repeated episodes lead to portal tract fibrosis - secondary biliary cirrhosis

Drug induced liver injury
- 10% of adverse drug reactions involve liver
- Predictable (dose related) or unpredictable (idiosyncratic)
- Hepatocellular or cholestatic

Alcoholic liver disease
- Common cause of acute and chronic liver disease
- Causes 3 forms of liver disease - Hepatic steatosis (fatty change in liver cells) alcoholic hepatitis and cirrhosis

Pathogenesis
- Diversion of metabolic pathways to metabolism of alcohol, production of acetylaldehyde which is hepatotoxic and stimulation of collagen synthesis -> fibrosis

SYSTEMATIC PATHOLOGY

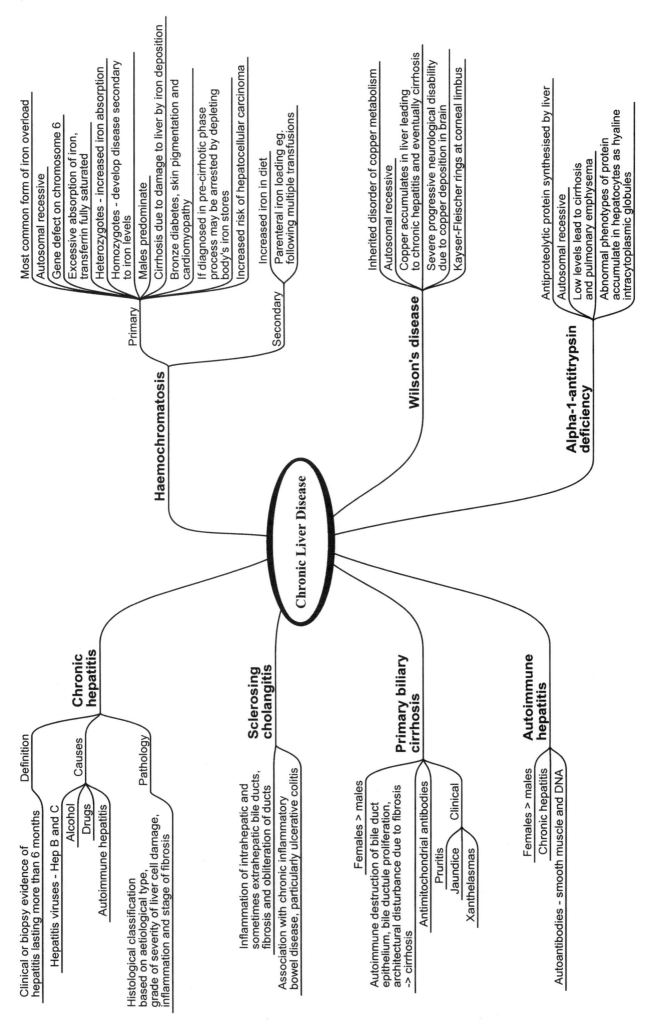

Chronic Liver Disease

Haemochromatosis

Primary
- Most common form of iron overload
- Autosomal recessive
- Gene defect on chromosome 6
- Excessive absorption of iron, transferrin fully saturated
- Heterozygotes - increased iron absorption
- Homozygotes - develop disease secondary to iron levels
- Males predominate
- Cirrhosis due to damage to liver by iron deposition
- Bronze diabetes, skin pigmentation and cardiomyopathy
- If diagnosed in pre-cirrhotic phase process may be arrested by depleting body's iron stores
- Increased risk of hepatocellular carcinoma

Secondary
- Increased iron in diet
- Parenteral iron loading eg. following multiple transfusions

Wilson's disease
- Inherited disorder of copper metabolism
- Autosomal recessive
- Copper accumulates in liver leading to chronic hepatitis and eventually cirrhosis
- Severe progressive neurological disability due to copper deposition in brain
- Kayser-Fleischer rings at corneal limbus

Alpha-1-antitrypsin deficiency
- Antiproteolytic protein synthesised by liver
- Autosomal recessive
- Low levels lead to cirrhosis and pulmonary emphysema
- Abnormal phenotypes of protein accumulate in hepatocytes as hyaline intracytoplasmic globules

Chronic hepatitis

Definition
- Clinical or biopsy evidence of hepatitis lasting more than 6 months

Causes
- Hepatitis viruses - Hep B and C
- Alcohol
- Drugs
- Autoimmune hepatitis

Pathology
- Histological classification based on aetiological type, grade of severity of liver cell damage, inflammation and stage of fibrosis

Sclerosing cholangitis
- Inflammation of intrahepatic and sometimes extrahepatic bile ducts, fibrosis and obliteration of ducts
- Association with chronic inflammatory bowel disease, particularly ulcerative colitis

Primary biliary cirrhosis
- Females > males
- Autoimmune destruction of bile duct epithelium, bile ductule proliferation, architectural disturbance due to fibrosis -> cirrhosis
- Antimitochondrial antibodies

Clinical
- Pruritis
- Jaundice
- Xanthelasmas

Autoimmune hepatitis
- Females > males
- Chronic hepatitis
- Autoantibodies - smooth muscle and DNA

SYSTEMATIC PATHOLOGY

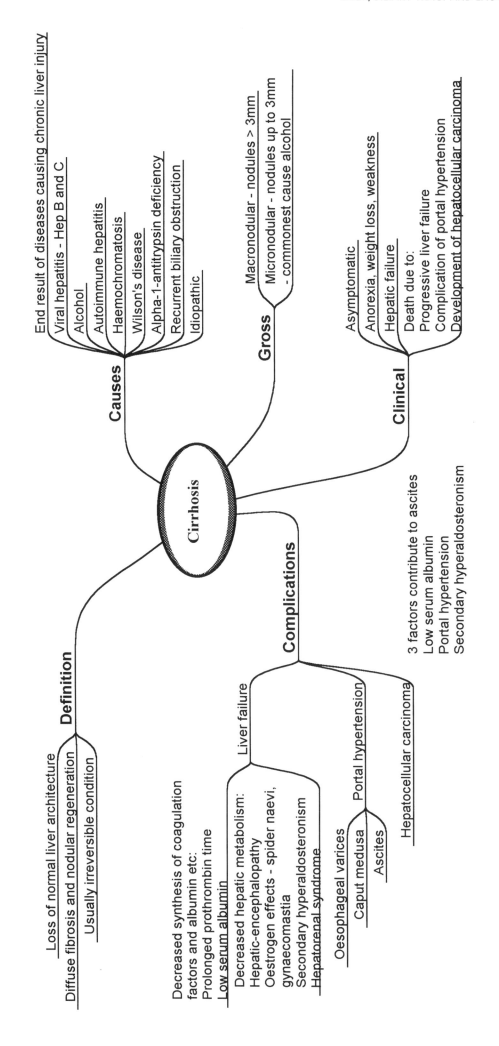

Cirrhosis

Causes
- End result of diseases causing chronic liver injury
- Viral hepatitis - Hep B and C
- Alcohol
- Autoimmune hepatitis
- Haemochromatosis
- Wilson's disease
- Alpha-1-antitrypsin deficiency
- Recurrent biliary obstruction
- Idiopathic

Gross
- Macronodular - nodules > 3mm
- Micronodular - nodules up to 3mm
  - commonest cause alcohol

Clinical
- Asymptomatic
- Anorexia, weight loss, weakness
- Hepatic failure
- Death due to:
- Progressive liver failure
- Complication of portal hypertension
- Development of hepatocellular carcinoma

Definition
- Loss of normal liver architecture
- Diffuse fibrosis and nodular regeneration
- Usually irreversible condition

Complications

Liver failure
- Decreased synthesis of coagulation factors and albumin etc:
- Prolonged prothrombin time
- Low serum albumin
- Decreased hepatic metabolism:
- Hepatic-encephalopathy
- Oestrogen effects - spider naevi, gynaecomastia
- Secondary hyperaldosteronism
- Hepatorenal syndrome

Portal hypertension
- Oesophageal varices
- Caput medusa
- Ascites

Hepatocellular carcinoma

3 factors contribute to ascites
Low serum albumin
Portal hypertension
Secondary hyperaldosteronism

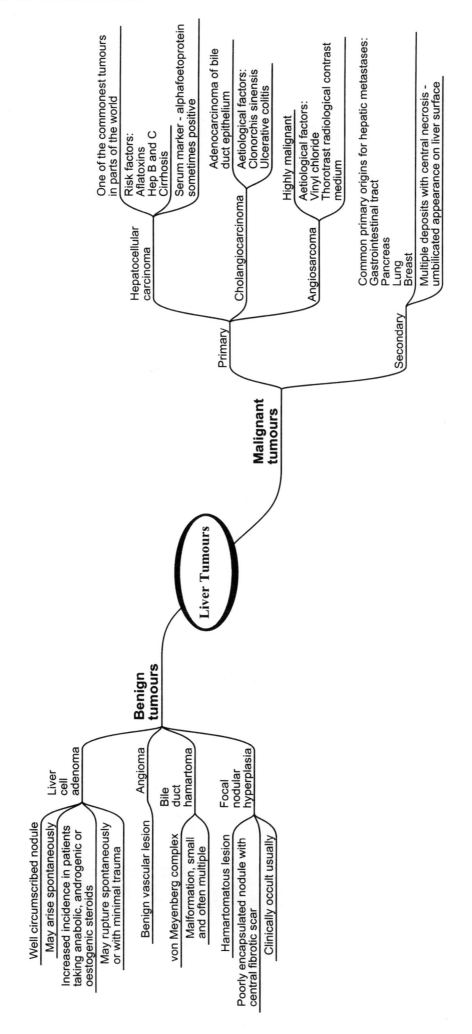

Liver Tumours

Benign tumours

Liver cell adenoma
- Well circumscribed nodule
- May arise spontaneously
- Increased incidence in patients taking anabolic, androgenic or oestogenic steroids
- May rupture spontaneously or with minimal trauma

Angioma
- Benign vascular lesion

Bile duct hamartoma
- von Meyenberg complex
- Malformation, small and often multiple

Focal nodular hyperplasia
- Hamartomatous lesion
- Poorly encapsulated nodule with central fibrotic scar
- Clinically occult usually

Malignant tumours

Primary

Hepatocellular carcinoma
- One of the commonest tumours in parts of the world
- Risk factors:
  Aflatoxins
  Hep B and C
  Cirrhosis
- Serum marker - alphafoetoprotein sometimes positive

Cholangiocarcinoma
- Adenocarcinoma of bile duct epithelium
- Aetiological factors:
  Clonorchis sinensis
  Ulcerative colitis

Angiosarcoma
- Highly malignant
- Aetiological factors:
  Vinyl chloride
  Thorotrast radiological contrast medium

Secondary
- Common primary origins for hepatic metastases:
  Gastrointestinal tract
  Pancreas
  Lung
  Breast
- Multiple deposits with central necrosis - umbilicated appearance on liver surface

SYSTEMATIC PATHOLOGY

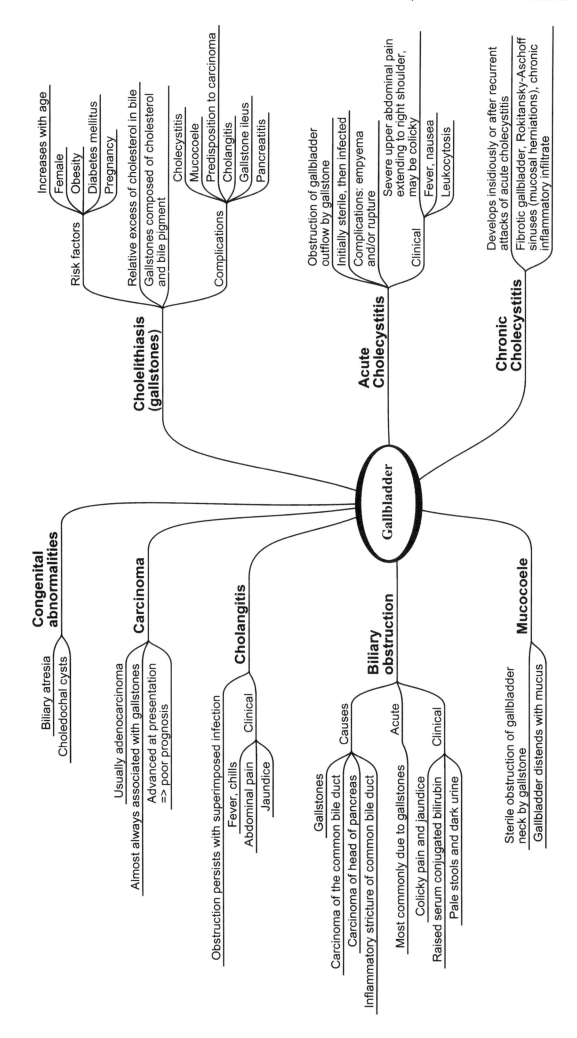

Gallbladder

Cholelithiasis (gallstones)
- Risk factors
  - Increases with age
  - Female
  - Obesity
  - Diabetes mellitus
  - Pregnancy
- Relative excess of cholesterol in bile
- Gallstones composed of cholesterol and bile pigment
- Complications
  - Cholecystitis
  - Mucocoele
  - Predisposition to carcinoma
  - Cholangitis
  - Gallstone ileus
  - Pancreatitis

Acute Cholecystitis
- Obstruction of gallbladder outflow by gallstone
- Initially sterile, then infected
- Complications: empyema and/or rupture
- Clinical
  - Severe upper abdominal pain extending to right shoulder, may be colicky
  - Fever, nausea
  - Leukocytosis

Chronic Cholecystitis
- Develops insidiously or after recurrent attacks of acute cholecystitis
- Fibrotic gallbladder, Rokitansky-Aschoff sinuses (mucosal herniations), chronic inflammatory infiltrate

Congenital abnormalities
- Biliary atresia
- Choledochal cysts

Carcinoma
- Usually adenocarcinoma
- Almost always associated with gallstones
- Advanced at presentation => poor prognosis

Cholangitis
- Obstruction persists with superimposed infection
- Clinical
  - Fever, chills
  - Abdominal pain
  - Jaundice

Biliary obstruction
- Causes
  - Gallstones
  - Carcinoma of the common bile duct
  - Carcinoma of head of pancreas
  - Inflammatory stricture of common bile duct
- Acute
  - Most commonly due to gallstones
- Clinical
  - Colicky pain and jaundice
  - Raised serum conjugated bilirubin
  - Pale stools and dark urine

Mucocoele
- Sterile obstruction of gallbladder neck by gallstone
- Gallbladder distends with mucus

SYSTEMATIC PATHOLOGY

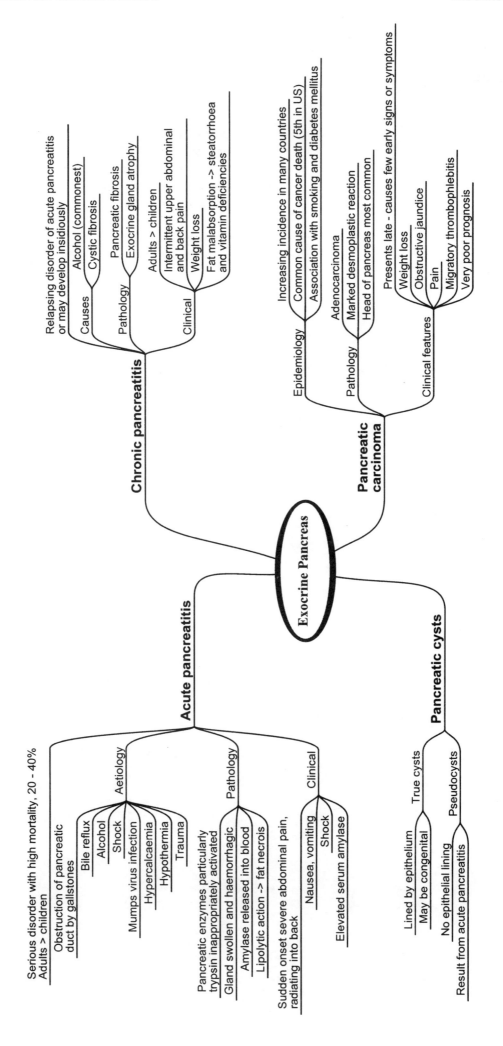

Exocrine Pancreas

Chronic pancreatitis

Relapsing disorder of acute pancreatitis or may develop insidiously

Causes
- Alcohol (commonest)
- Cystic fibrosis

Pathology
- Pancreatic fibrosis
- Exocrine gland atrophy

Clinical
- Adults > children
- Intermittent upper abdominal and back pain
- Weight loss
- Fat malabsorption -> steatorrhoea and vitamin deficiencies

Pancreatic carcinoma

Epidemiology
- Increasing incidence in many countries
- Common cause of cancer death (5th in US)
- Association with smoking and diabetes mellitus

Pathology
- Adenocarcinoma
- Marked desmoplastic reaction
- Head of pancreas most common

Clinical features
- Presents late - causes few early signs or symptoms
- Weight loss
- Obstructive jaundice
- Pain
- Migratory thrombophlebitis
- Very poor prognosis

Acute pancreatitis

Serious disorder with high mortality, 20 - 40%
Adults > children
Obstruction of pancreatic duct by gallstones

Aetiology
- Bile reflux
- Alcohol
- Shock
- Mumps virus infection
- Hypercalcaemia
- Hypothermia
- Trauma

Pathology
- Pancreatic enzymes particularly trypsin inappropriately activated
- Gland swollen and haemorrhagic
- Amylase released into blood
- Lipolytic action -> fat necrosis

Clinical
- Sudden onset severe abdominal pain, radiating into back
- Nausea, vomiting
- Shock
- Elevated serum amylase

Pancreatic cysts

True cysts
- Lined by epithelium
- May be congenital

Pseudocysts
- No epithelial lining
- Result from acute pancreatitis

ENDOCRINE SYSTEM

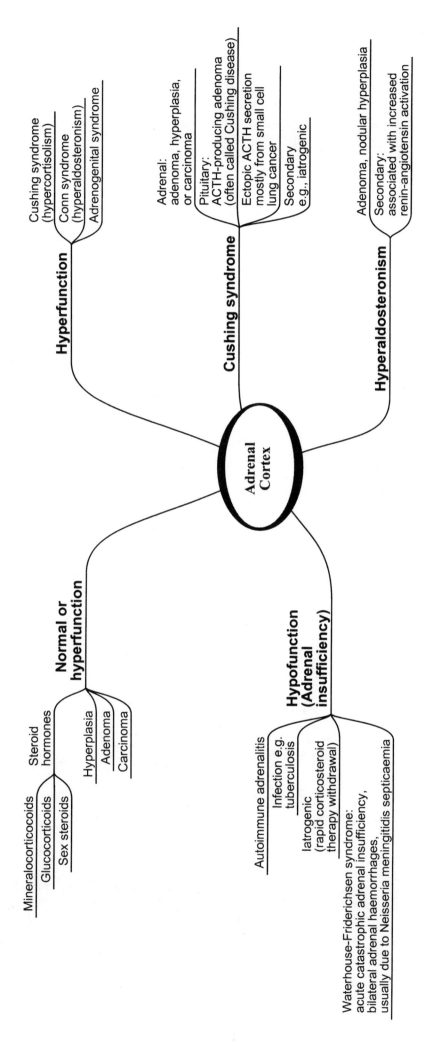

Adrenal Cortex

Hyperfunction

- Cushing syndrome (hypercortisolism)
- Conn syndrome (hyperaldosteronism)
- Adrenogenital syndrome

Cushing syndrome

- Adrenal: adenoma, hyperplasia, or carcinoma
- Pituitary: ACTH-producing adenoma (often called Cushing disease)
- Ectopic ACTH secretion mostly from small cell lung cancer
- Secondary e.g., iatrogenic

Hyperaldosteronism

- Adenoma, nodular hyperplasia
- Secondary: associated with increased renin-angiotensin activation

Normal or hyperfunction

- Steroid hormones
  - Mineralocorticoids
  - Glucocorticoids
  - Sex steroids
- Hyperplasia
- Adenoma
- Carcinoma

Hypofunction (Adrenal insufficiency)

- Autoimmune adrenalitis
- Infection e.g. tuberculosis
- Iatrogenic (rapid corticosteroid therapy withdrawal)
- Waterhouse-Friderichsen syndrome: acute catastrophic adrenal insufficiency, bilateral adrenal haemorrhages, usually due to Neisseria meningitidis septicaemia

SYSTEMATIC PATHOLOGY

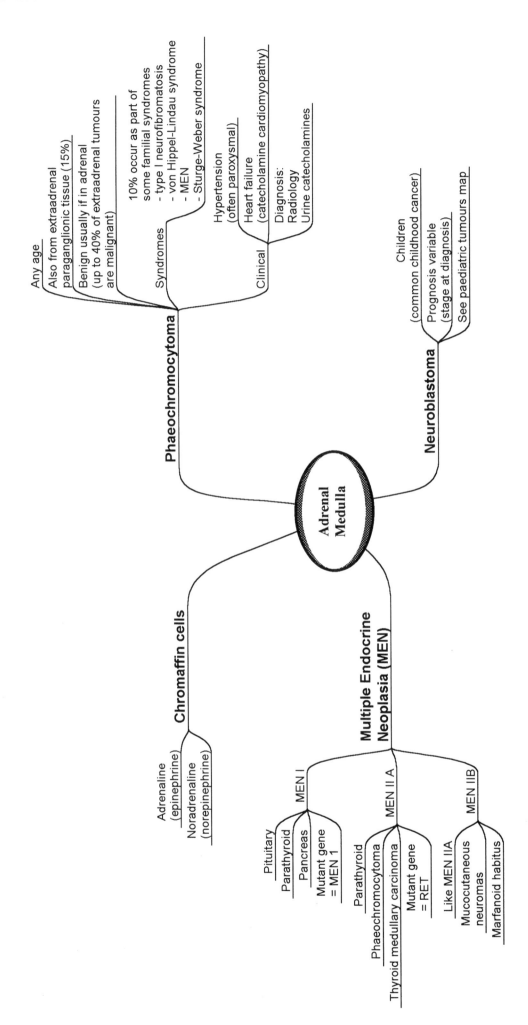

Adrenal Medulla

Phaeochromocytoma

- Any age
- Also from extraadrenal paraganglionic tissue (15%)
- Benign usually if in adrenal (up to 40% of extraadrenal tumours are malignant)
- Syndromes
  - 10% occur as part of some familial syndromes
    - type I neurofibromatosis
    - von Hippel–Lindau syndrome
    - MEN
    - Sturge–Weber syndrome
- Clinical
  - Hypertension (often paroxysmal)
  - Heart failure (catecholamine cardiomyopathy)
  - Diagnosis: Radiology Urine catecholamines

Neuroblastoma

- Children (common childhood cancer)
- Prognosis variable (stage at diagnosis)
- See paediatric tumours map

Chromaffin cells

- Adrenaline (epinephrine)
- Noradrenaline (norepinephrine)

Multiple Endocrine Neoplasia (MEN)

- MEN I
  - Pituitary
  - Parathyroid
  - Pancreas
  - Mutant gene = MEN 1
- MEN II A
  - Parathyroid
  - Phaeochromocytoma
  - Thyroid medullary carcinoma
  - Mutant gene = RET
- MEN IIB
  - Like MEN IIA
  - Mucocutaneous neuromas
  - Marfanoid habitus

SYSTEMATIC PATHOLOGY

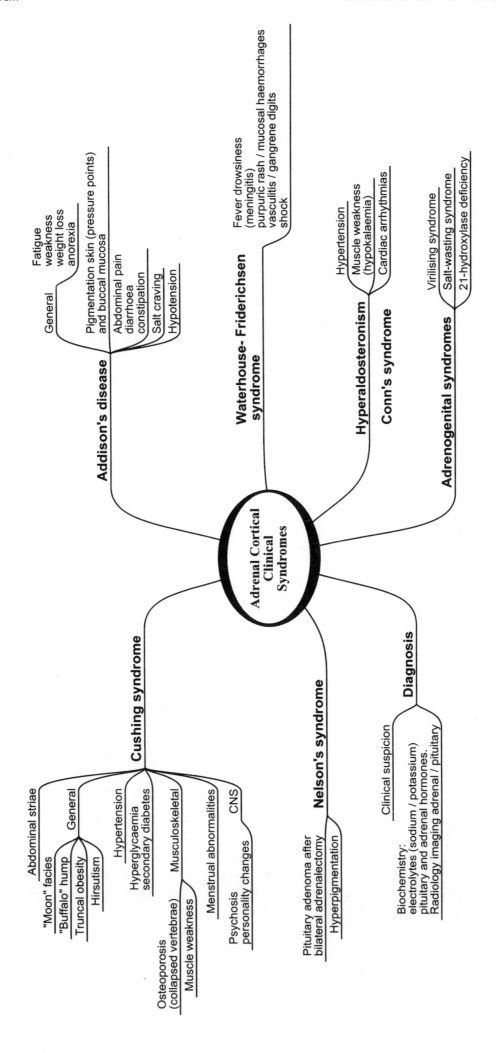

Adrenal Cortical Clinical Syndromes

Addison's disease

General
- Fatigue
- weakness
- weight loss
- anorexia

- Pigmentation skin (pressure points) and buccal mucosa
- Abdominal pain
- diarrhoea
- constipation
- Salt craving
- Hypotension

Waterhouse-Friderichsen syndrome
- Fever drowsiness (meningitis)
- purpuric rash / mucosal haemorrhages
- vasculitis / gangrene digits
- shock

Hyperaldosteronism

Conn's syndrome
- Hypertension
- Muscle weakness (hypokalaemia)
- Cardiac arrhythmias

Adrenogenital syndromes
- Virilising syndrome
- Salt-wasting syndrome
- 21-hydroxylase deficiency

Cushing syndrome
- Abdominal striae

General
- "Moon" facies
- "Buffalo" hump
- Truncal obesity
- Hirsutism

- Hypertension
- Hyperglycaemia secondary diabetes

Musculoskeletal
- Osteoporosis (collapsed vertebrae)
- Muscle weakness

- Menstrual abnormalities

CNS
- Psychosis
- personality changes

Nelson's syndrome
- Pituitary adenoma after bilateral adrenalectomy
- Hyperpigmentation

Diagnosis
- Clinical suspicion
- Biochemistry: electrolytes (sodium / potassium) pituitary and adrenal hormones.
- Radiology imaging adrenal / pituitary

SYSTEMATIC PATHOLOGY

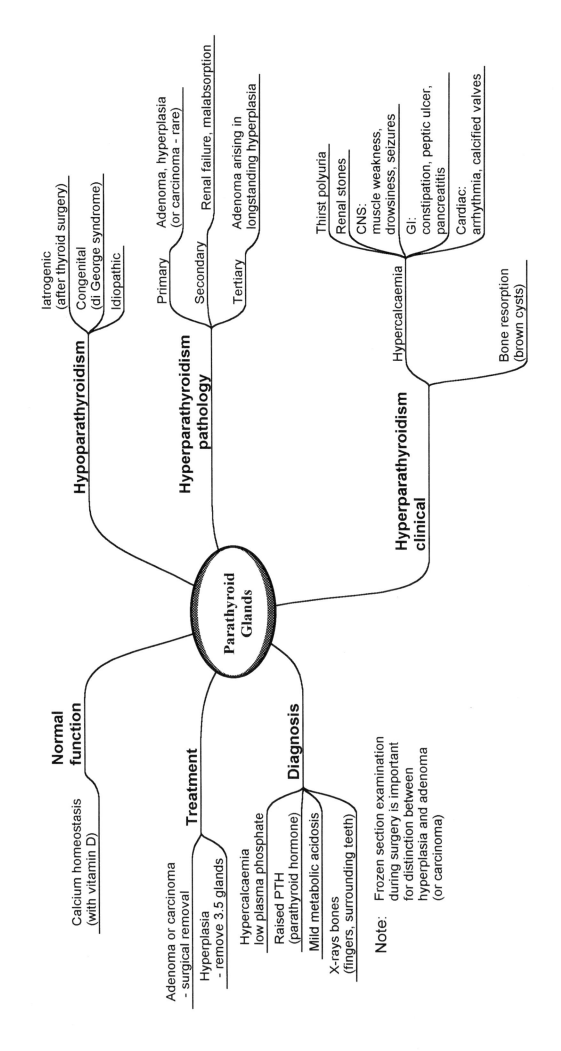

Parathyroid Glands

Hypoparathyroidism
- Iatrogenic (after thyroid surgery)
- Congenital (di George syndrome)
- Idiopathic

Hyperparathyroidism pathology
- Primary — Adenoma, hyperplasia (or carcinoma - rare)
- Secondary — Renal failure, malabsorption
- Tertiary — Adenoma arising in longstanding hyperplasia

Hyperparathyroidism clinical
- Hypercalcaemia
  - Thirst polyuria
  - Renal stones
  - CNS: muscle weakness, drowsiness, seizures
  - GI: constipation, peptic ulcer, pancreatitis
  - Cardiac: arrhythmia, calcified valves
- Bone resorption (brown cysts)

Normal function
- Calcium homeostasis (with vitamin D)

Treatment
- Adenoma or carcinoma - surgical removal
- Hyperplasia - remove 3.5 glands

Diagnosis
- Hypercalcaemia low plasma phosphate
- Raised PTH (parathyroid hormone)
- Mild metabolic acidosis
- X-rays bones (fingers, surrounding teeth)

Note: Frozen section examination during surgery is important for distinction between hyperplasia and adenoma (or carcinoma)

SYSTEMATIC PATHOLOGY

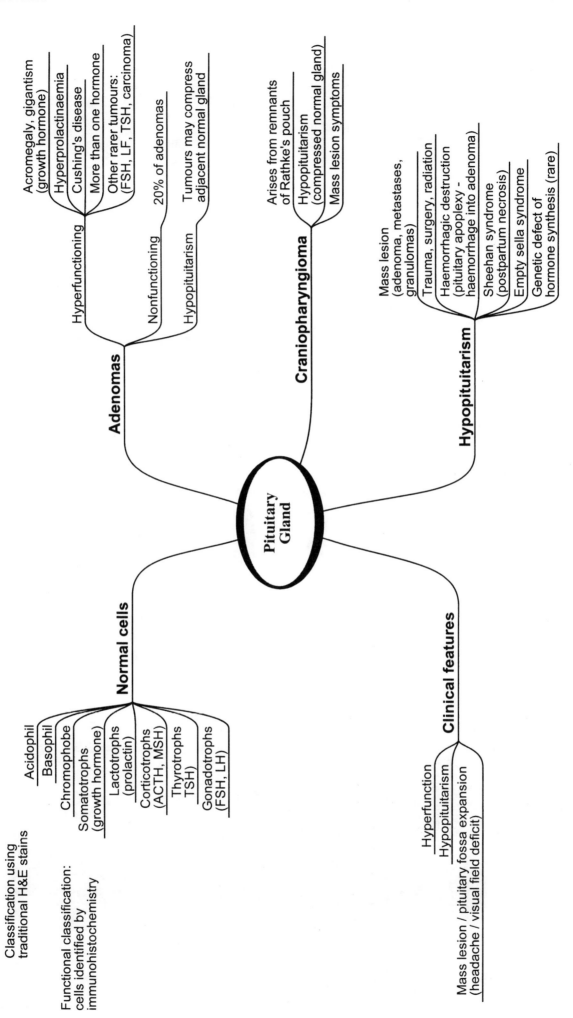

Pituitary Gland

Adenomas

Hyperfunctioning
- Acromegaly, gigantism (growth hormone)
- Hyperprolactinaemia
- Cushing's disease
- More than one hormone
- Other rarer tumours: (FSH, LF, TSH, carcinoma)

Nonfunctioning
- 20% of adenomas

Hypopituitarism
- Tumours may compress adjacent normal gland

Craniopharyngioma
- Arises from remnants of Rathke's pouch
- Hypopituitarism (compressed normal gland)
- Mass lesion symptoms

Hypopituitarism
- Mass lesion (adenoma, metastases, granulomas)
- Trauma, surgery, radiation
- Haemorrhagic destruction (pituitary apoplexy - haemorrhage into adenoma)
- Sheehan syndrome (postpartum necrosis)
- Empty sella syndrome
- Genetic defect of hormone synthesis (rare)

Normal cells

Classification using traditional H&E stains
- Acidophil
- Basophil
- Chromophobe

Functional classification: cells identified by immunohistochemistry
- Somatotrophs (growth hormone)
- Lactotrophs (prolactin)
- Corticotrophs (ACTH, MSH)
- Thyrotrophs (TSH)
- Gonadotrophs (FSH, LH)

Clinical features
- Hyperfunction
- Hypopituitarism
- Mass lesion / pituitary fossa expansion (headache / visual field deficit)

SYSTEMATIC PATHOLOGY

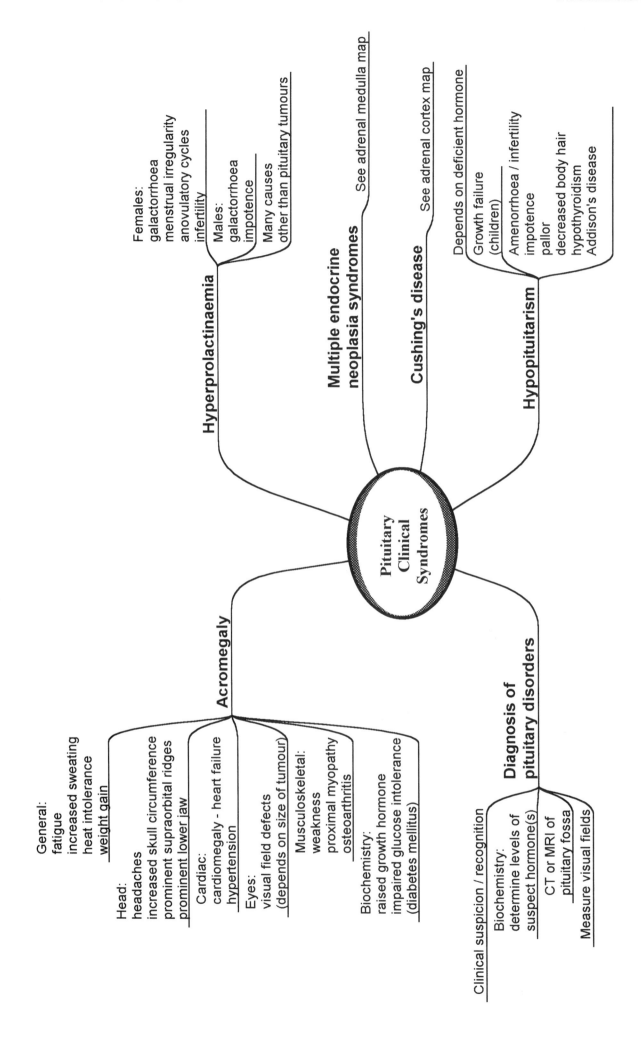

Pituitary Clinical Syndromes

Hyperprolactinaemia

Females:
galactorrhoea
menstrual irregularity
anovulatory cycles
infertility

Males:
galactorrhoea
impotence

Many causes
other than pituitary tumours

Multiple endocrine neoplasia syndromes

See adrenal medulla map

Cushing's disease

See adrenal cortex map

Hypopituitarism

Depends on deficient hormone

Growth failure
(children)

Amenorrhoea / infertility
impotence
pallor
decreased body hair
hypothyroidism
Addison's disease

Acromegaly

General:
fatigue
increased sweating
heat intolerance
weight gain

Head:
headaches
increased skull circumference
prominent supraorbital ridges
prominent lower jaw

Cardiac:
cardiomegaly - heart failure
hypertension

Eyes:
visual field defects
(depends on size of tumour)

Musculoskeletal:
weakness
proximal myopathy
osteoarthritis

Biochemistry:
raised growth hormone
impaired glucose intolerance
(diabetes mellitus)

Diagnosis of pituitary disorders

Clinical suspicion / recognition

Biochemistry:
determine levels of
suspect hormone(s)

CT or MRI of
pituitary fossa

Measure visual fields

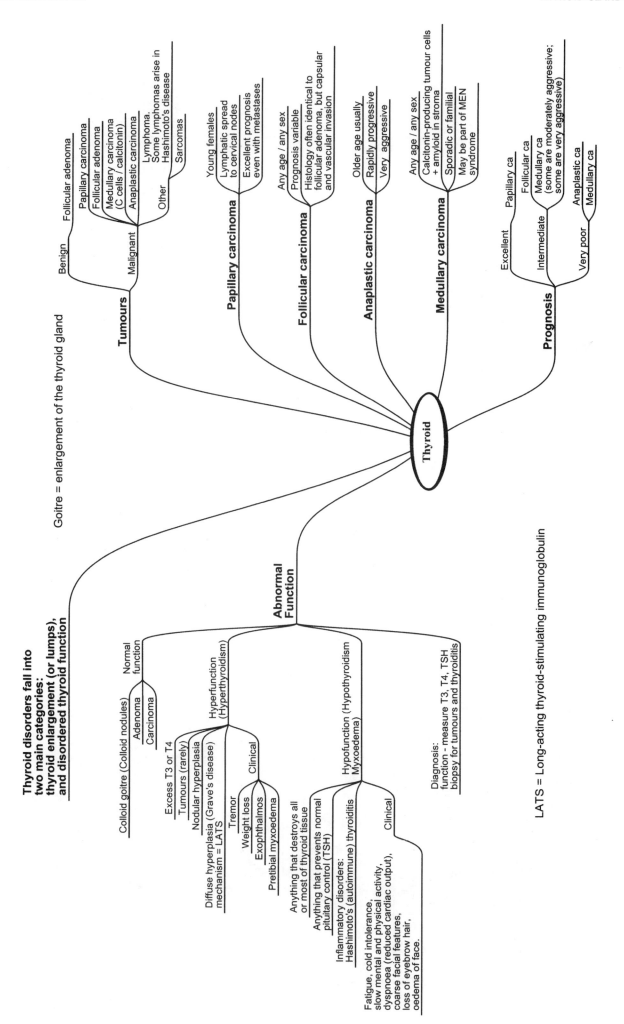

Thyroid disorders fall into two main categories: thyroid enlargement (or lumps), and disordered thyroid function

Goitre = enlargement of the thyroid gland

Tumours

Benign — Follicular adenoma

Malignant — Papillary carcinoma
— Follicular adenoma
— Medullary carcinoma (C cells / calcitonin)
— Anaplastic carcinoma
— Lymphoma. Some lymphomas arise in Hashimoto's disease
Other — Sarcomas

Papillary carcinoma
— Young females
— Lymphatic spread to cervical nodes
— Excellent prognosis even with metastases

Follicular carcinoma
— Any age / any sex
— Prognosis variable
— Histology often identical to follicular adenoma, but capsular and vascular invasion

Anaplastic carcinoma
— Older age usually
— Rapidly progressive
— Very aggressive

Medullary carcinoma
— Any age / any sex
— Calcitonin-producing tumour cells + amyloid in stroma
— Sporadic or familial
— May be part of MEN syndrome

Prognosis
Excellent — Papillary ca
Intermediate — Follicular ca
— Medullary ca (some are moderately aggressive; some are very aggressive)
Very poor — Anaplastic ca
— Medullary ca

Thyroid

Abnormal Function

Normal function — Colloid goitre (Colloid nodules)
— Adenoma
— Carcinoma

Hyperfunction (Hyperthyroidism)
— Excess T3 or T4
— Tumours (rarely)
— Nodular hyperplasia
— Diffuse hyperplasia (Grave's disease) mechanism = LATS

Clinical — Tremor
— Weight loss
— Exophthalmos
— Pretibial myxoedema

Hypofunction (Hypothyroidism) Myxoedema
— Anything that destroys all or most of thyroid tissue
— Anything that prevents normal pituitary control (TSH)
— Inflammatory disorders: Hashimoto's (autoimmune) thyroiditis

Clinical — Fatigue, cold intolerance, slow mental and physical activity, dyspnoea (reduced cardiac output), coarse facial features, loss of eyebrow hair, oedema of face.

Diagnosis: function - measure T3, T4, TSH biopsy for tumours and thyroiditis

LATS = Long-acting thyroid-stimulating immunoglobulin

SYSTEMATIC PATHOLOGY

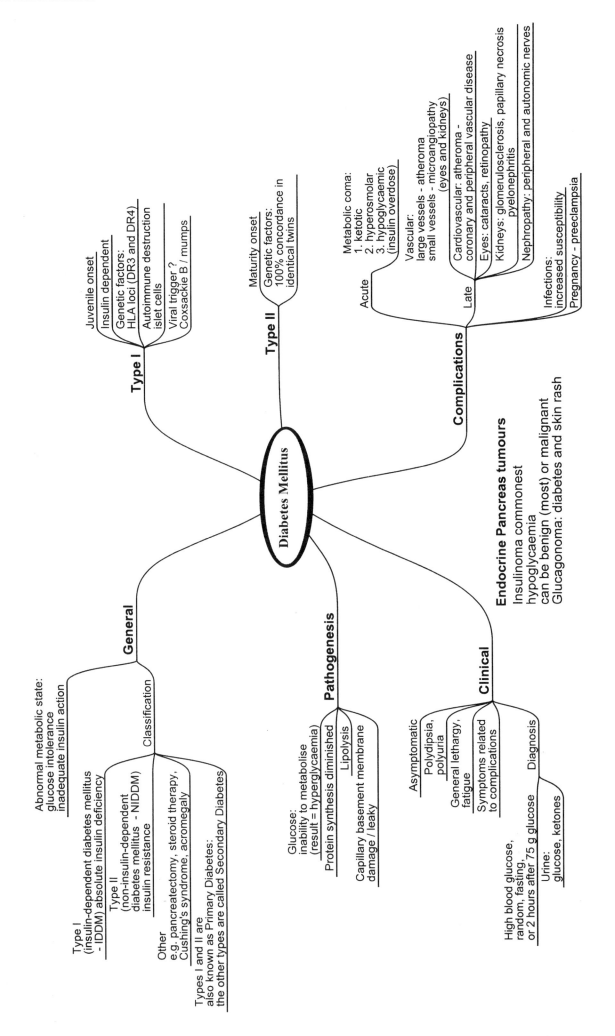

Diabetes Mellitus

Type I
- Juvenile onset
- Insulin dependent
- Genetic factors: HLA loci (DR3 and DR4)
- Autoimmune destruction islet cells
- Viral trigger ? Coxsackie B / mumps

Type II
- Maturity onset
- Genetic factors: 100% concordance in identical twins

Complications

Acute
- Metabolic coma:
  1. ketotic
  2. hyperosmolar
  3. hypoglycaemic (insulin overdose)

Late
- Vascular:
  large vessels - atheroma
  small vessels - microangiopathy (eyes and kidneys)
- Cardiovascular: atheroma - coronary and peripheral vascular disease
- Eyes: cataracts, retinopathy
- Kidneys: glomerulosclerosis, papillary necrosis pyelonephritis
- Nephropathy: peripheral and autonomic nerves
- Infections: increased susceptibility
- Pregnancy - preeclampsia

General

Abnormal metabolic state: glucose intolerance inadequate insulin action

Classification
- Type I (insulin-dependent diabetes mellitus - IDDM) absolute insulin deficiency
- Type II (non-insulin-dependent diabetes mellitus - NIDDM) insulin resistance
- Other
  e.g. pancreatectomy, steroid therapy, Cushing's syndrome, acromegaly

Types I and II are also known as Primary Diabetes: the other types are called Secondary Diabetes

Pathogenesis
- Glucose: inability to metabolise (result = hyperglycaemia)
- Protein synthesis diminished
- Lipolysis
- Capillary basement membrane damage / leaky

Clinical
- Asymptomatic
- Polydipsia, polyuria
- General lethargy, fatigue
- Symptoms related to complications

Diagnosis
- High blood glucose, random, fasting, or 2 hours after 75 g glucose
- Urine: glucose, ketones

Endocrine Pancreas tumours
- Insulinoma commonest hypoglycaemia can be benign (most) or malignant
- Glucagonoma: diabetes and skin rash

KIDNEYS AND URINARY TRACT

SYSTEMATIC PATHOLOGY

SYSTEMATIC PATHOLOGY

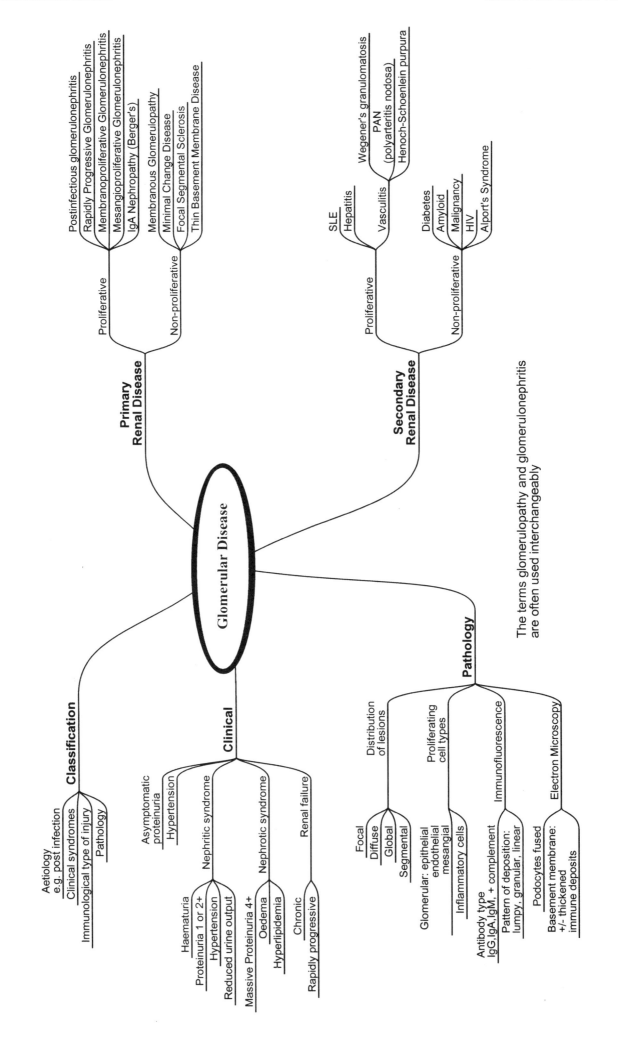

The terms glomerulopathy and glomerulonephritis are often used interchangeably

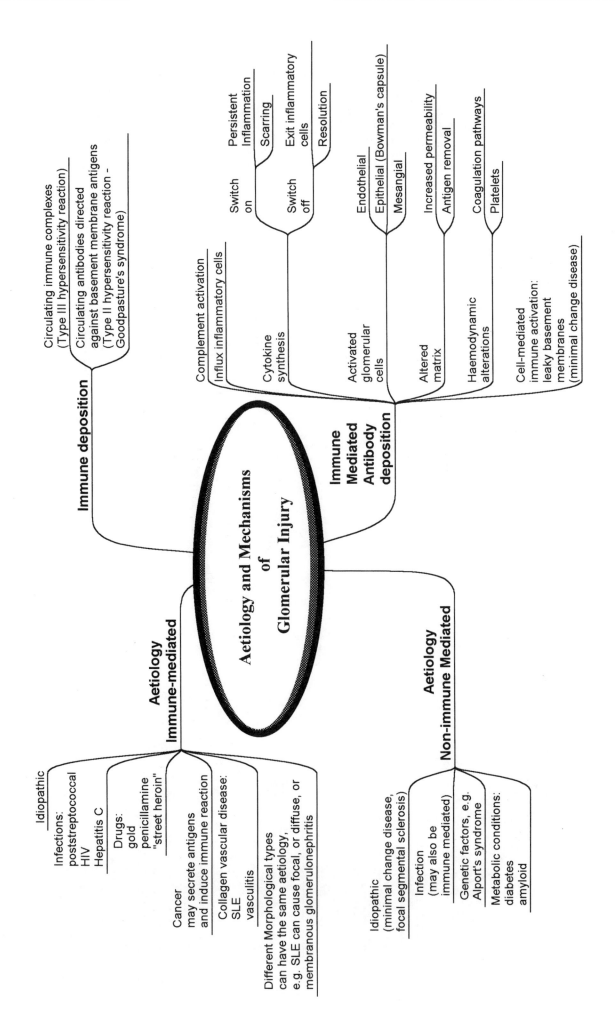

SYSTEMATIC PATHOLOGY

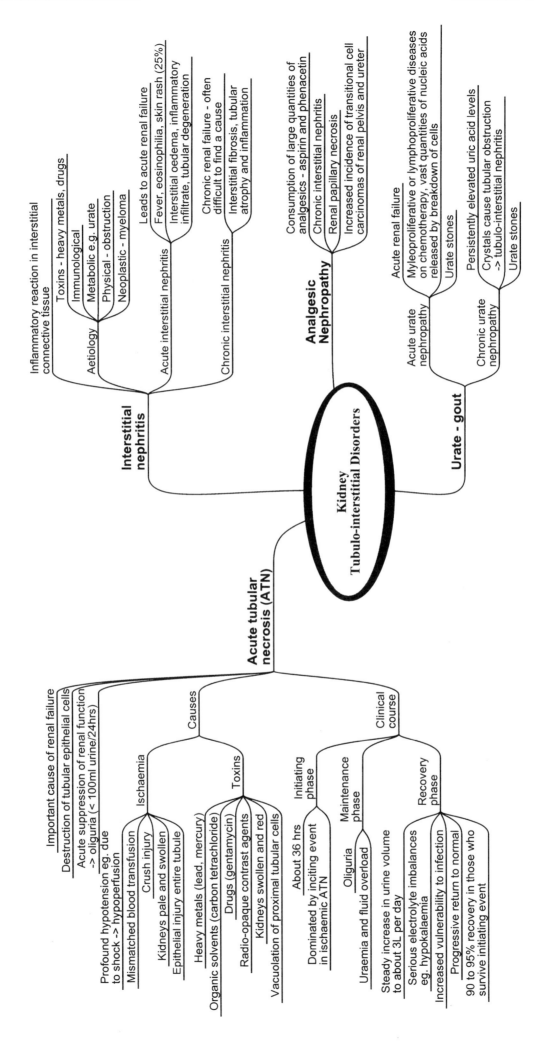

Kidney Tubulo-interstitial Disorders

Interstitial nephritis

Aetiology
- Inflammatory reaction in interstitial connective tissue
- Toxins - heavy metals, drugs
- Immunological
- Metabolic e.g. urate
- Physical - obstruction
- Neoplastic - myeloma

Acute interstitial nephritis
- Leads to acute renal failure
- Fever, eosinophilia, skin rash (25%)
- Interstitial oedema, inflammatory infiltrate, tubular degeneration

Chronic interstitial nephritis
- Chronic renal failure - often difficult to find a cause
- Interstitial fibrosis, tubular atrophy and inflammation

Analgesic Nephropathy
- Consumption of large quantities of analgesics - aspirin and phenacetin
- Chronic interstitial nephritis
- Renal papillary necrosis
- Increased incidence of transitional cell carcinomas of renal pelvis and ureter

Urate - gout

Acute urate nephropathy
- Acute renal failure
- Myeloproliferative or lymphoproliferative diseases on chemotherapy, vast quantities of nucleic acids released by breakdown of cells
- Urate stones

Chronic urate nephropathy
- Persistently elevated uric acid levels
- Crystals cause tubular obstruction -> tubulo-interstitial nephritis
- Urate stones

Acute tubular necrosis (ATN)

Causes
- Important cause of renal failure
- Destruction of tubular epithelial cells
- Acute suppression of renal function -> oliguria (< 100ml urine/24hrs)

Ischaemia
- Profound hypotension eg. due to shock -> hypoperfusion
- Mismatched blood transfusion
- Crush injury
- Kidneys pale and swollen
- Epithelial injury entire tubule

Toxins
- Heavy metals (lead, mercury)
- Organic solvents (carbon tetrachloride)
- Drugs (gentamicin)
- Radio-opaque contrast agents
- Kidneys swollen and red
- Vacuolation of proximal tubular cells

Clinical course

Initiating phase
- About 36 hrs
- Dominated by inciting event in ischaemic ATN

Maintenance phase
- Oliguria
- Uraemia and fluid overload

Recovery phase
- Steady increase in urine volume to about 3L per day
- Serious electrolyte imbalances eg. hypokalaemia
- Increased vulnerability to infection
- Progressive return to normal
- 90 to 95% recovery in those who survive initiating event

SYSTEMATIC PATHOLOGY

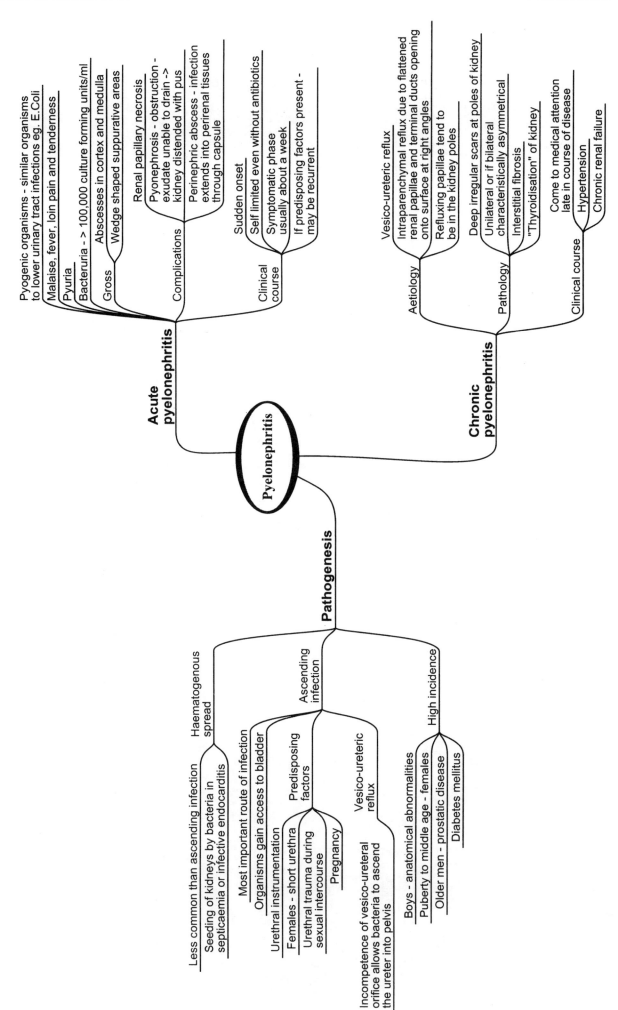

Pyelonephritis

Acute pyelonephritis

Pyogenic organisms - similar organisms to lower urinary tract infections eg. E.Coli

Malaise, fever, loin pain and tenderness

Pyuria

Bacteruria - > 100,000 culture forming units/ml

Gross
- Abscesses in cortex and medulla
- Wedge shaped suppurative areas

Complications
- Renal papillary necrosis
- Pyonephrosis - obstruction - exudate unable to drain -> kidney distended with pus
- Perinephric abscess - infection extends into perirenal tissues through capsule

Clinical course
- Sudden onset
- Self limited even without antibiotics
- Symptomatic phase usually about a week
- If predisposing factors present - may be recurrent

Chronic pyelonephritis

Aetiology
- Vesico-ureteric reflux
- Intraparenchymal reflux due to flattened renal papillae and terminal ducts opening onto surface at right angles
- Refluxing papillae tend to be in the kidney poles

Pathology
- Deep irregular scars at poles of kidney
- Unilateral or if bilateral characteristically asymmetrical
- Interstitial fibrosis
- "Thyroidisation" of kidney

Clinical course
- Come to medical attention late in course of disease
- Hypertension
- Chronic renal failure

Pathogenesis

Haematogenous spread
- Less common than ascending infection
- Seeding of kidneys by bacteria in septicaemia or infective endocarditis

Ascending infection
- Most important route of infection
- Organisms gain access to bladder
- Urethral instrumentation

Predisposing factors
- Females - short urethra
- Urethral trauma during sexual intercourse
- Pregnancy

Vesico-ureteric reflux
- Incompetence of vesico-ureteral orifice allows bacteria to ascend the ureter into pelvis

High incidence
- Boys - anatomical abnormalities
- Puberty to middle age - females
- Older men - prostatic disease
- Diabetes mellitus

SYSTEMATIC PATHOLOGY

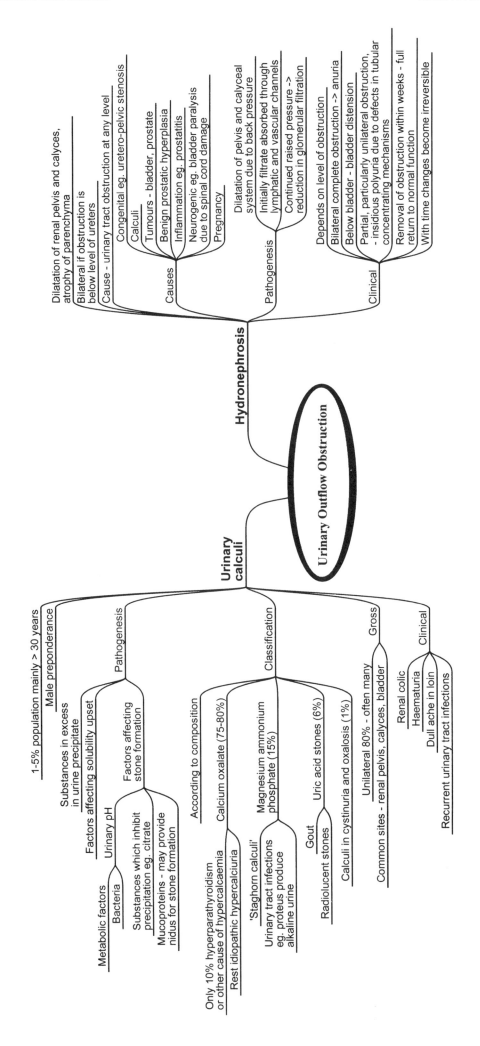

Urinary Outflow Obstruction

Hydronephrosis

Causes
- Dilatation of renal pelvis and calyces, atrophy of parenchyma
- Bilateral if obstruction is below level of ureters
- Cause - urinary tract obstruction at any level
  - Congenital eg. uretero-pelvic stenosis
  - Calculi
  - Tumours - bladder, prostate
  - Benign prostatic hyperplasia
  - Inflammation eg. prostatitis
  - Neurogenic eg. bladder paralysis due to spinal cord damage
  - Pregnancy

Pathogenesis
- Dilatation of pelvis and calyceal system due to back pressure
- Initially filtrate absorbed through lymphatic and vascular channels
- Continued raised pressure -> reduction in glomerular filtration

Clinical
- Depends on level of obstruction
- Bilateral complete obstruction -> anuria
- Below bladder - bladder distension
- Partial, particularly unilateral obstruction, - insidious polyuria due to defects in tubular concentrating mechanisms
- Removal of obstruction within weeks - full return to normal function
- With time changes become irreversible

Urinary calculi

Pathogenesis
- 1-5% population mainly > 30 years
- Male preponderance
- Substances in excess in urine precipitate
- Factors affecting solubility upset
  - Urinary pH
  - Factors affecting stone formation
    - Metabolic factors
    - Bacteria
    - Substances which inhibit precipitation eg. citrate
    - Mucoproteins - may provide nidus for stone formation
- Only 10% hyperparathyroidism or other cause of hypercalcaemia
- Rest idiopathic hypercalciuria

Classification
- According to composition
- Calcium oxalate (75-80%)
- Magnesium ammonium phosphate (15%)
  - 'Staghorn calculi'
  - Urinary tract infections eg. proteus produce alkaline urine
- Uric acid stones (6%)
  - Gout
  - Radiolucent stones
- Calculi in cystinuria and oxalosis (1%)

Gross
- Unilateral 80% - often many
- Common sites - renal pelvis, calyces, bladder

Clinical
- Renal colic
- Haematuria
- Dull ache in loin
- Recurrent urinary tract infections

SYSTEMATIC PATHOLOGY

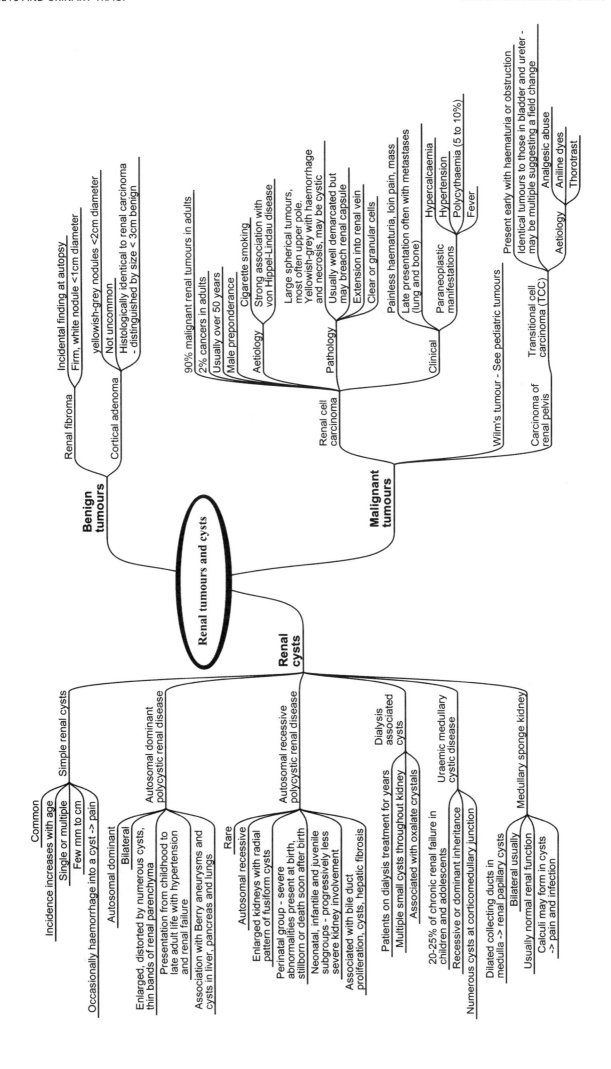

Renal tumours and cysts

Benign tumours

Renal fibroma
— Incidental finding at autopsy
— Firm, white nodule <1cm diameter

Cortical adenoma
— yellowish-grey nodules <2cm diameter
— Not uncommon
— Histologically identical to renal carcinoma - distinguished by size < 3cm benign

Malignant tumours

Renal cell carcinoma
— 90% malignant renal tumours in adults
— 2% cancers in adults
— Usually over 50 years
— Male preponderance
— Aetiology
  — Cigarette smoking
  — Strong association with von Hippel-Lindau disease
— Pathology
  — Large spherical tumours, most often upper pole.
  — Yellowish-grey with haemorrhage and necrosis, may be cystic
  — Usually well demarcated but may breach renal capsule
  — Extension into renal vein
  — Clear or granular cells
— Clinical
  — Painless haematuria, loin pain, mass
  — Late presentation often with metastases (lung and bone)
  — Paraneoplastic manifestations
    — Hypercalcaemia
    — Hypertension
    — Polycythaemia (5 to 10%)
    — Fever

Wilm's tumour - See pediatric tumours

Carcinoma of renal pelvis
— Present early with haematuria or obstruction
— Identical tumours to those in bladder and ureter - may be multiple suggesting a field change
— Transitional cell carcinoma (TCC)
— Aetiology
  — Analgesic abuse
  — Aniline dyes
  — Thorotrast

Renal cysts

Simple renal cysts
— Common
— Incidence increases with age
— Single or multiple
— Few mm to cm
— Occasionally haemorrhage into a cyst -> pain

Autosomal dominant polycystic renal disease
— Autosomal dominant
— Bilateral
— Enlarged, distorted by numerous cysts, thin bands of renal parenchyma
— Presentation from childhood to late adult life with hypertension and renal failure
— Association with Berry aneurysms and cysts in liver, pancreas and lungs

Autosomal recessive polycystic renal disease
— Rare
— Autosomal recessive
— Enlarged kidneys with radial pattern of fusiform cysts
— Perinatal group - severe abnormalities present at birth, stillborn or death soon after birth
— Neonatal, infantile and juvenile subgroups - progressively less severe kidney involvement
— Associated with bile duct proliferation, cysts, hepatic fibrosis

Dialysis associated cysts
— Patients on dialysis treatment for years
— Multiple small cysts throughout kidney
— Associated with oxalate crystals

Uraemic medullary cystic disease
— 20-25% of chronic renal failure in children and adolescents
— Recessive or dominant inheritance
— Numerous cysts at corticomedullary junction

Medullary sponge kidney
— Dilated collecting ducts in medulla -> renal papillary cysts
— Bilateral usually
— Usually normal renal function
— Calculi may form in cysts -> pain and infection

SYSTEMATIC PATHOLOGY

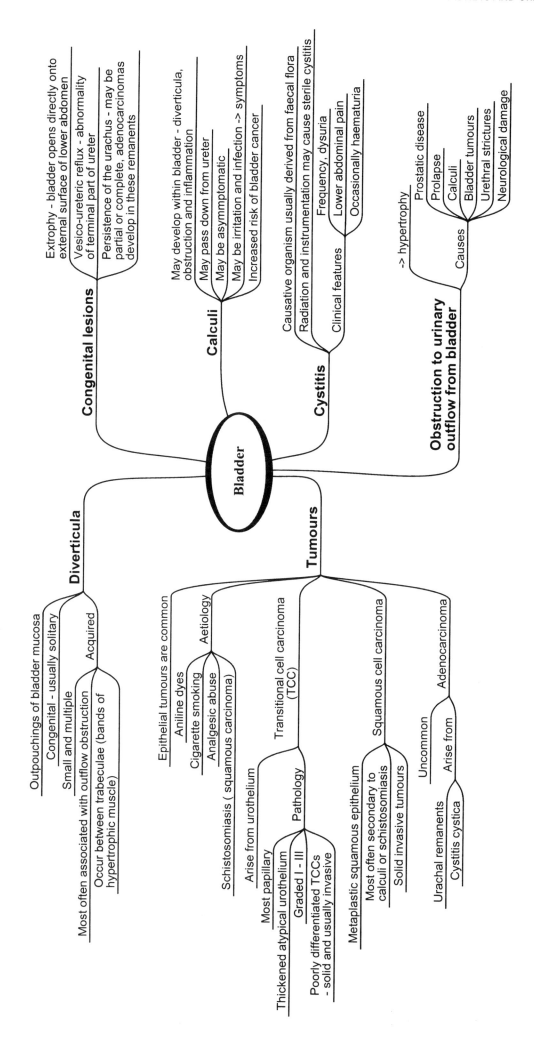

Bladder

Congenital lesions
- Extrophy - bladder opens directly onto external surface of lower abdomen
- Vesico-ureteric reflux - abnormality of terminal part of ureter
- Persistence of the urachus - may be partial or complete, adenocarcinomas develop in these remenants

Calculi
- May develop within bladder - diverticula, obstruction and inflammation
- May pass down from ureter
- May be asymmptomatic
- May be irritation and infection -> symptoms
- Increased risk of bladder cancer

Cystitis
- Causative organism usually derived from faecal flora
- Radiation and instrumentation may cause sterile cystitis
- Clinical features
  - Frequency, dysuria
  - Lower abdominal pain
  - Occasionally haematuria

Obstruction to urinary outflow from bladder
- -> hypertrophy
- Causes
  - Prostatic disease
  - Prolapse
  - Calculi
  - Bladder tumours
  - Urethral strictures
  - Neurological damage

Diverticula
- Outpouchings of bladder mucosa
- Congenital - usually solitary
- Small and multiple
  - Acquired
    - Most often associated with outflow obstruction
    - Occur between trabeculae (bands of hypertrophic muscle)

Tumours
- Epithelial tumours are common
- Aetiology
  - Aniline dyes
  - Cigarette smoking
  - Analgesic abuse
  - Schistosomiasis (squamous carcinoma)
- Transitional cell carcinoma (TCC)
  - Pathology
    - Arise from urothelium
    - Most papillary
    - Graded I - III
    - Thickened atypical urothelium
    - Poorly differentiated TCCs - solid and usually invasive
- Squamous cell carcinoma
  - Metaplastic squamous epithelium
  - Most often secondary to calculi or schistosomiasis
  - Solid invasive tumours
- Adenocarcinoma
  - Uncommon
  - Arise from
    - Urachal remanents
    - Cystitis cystica

MALE GENITAL TRACT

SYSTEMATIC PATHOLOGY

SYSTEMATIC PATHOLOGY

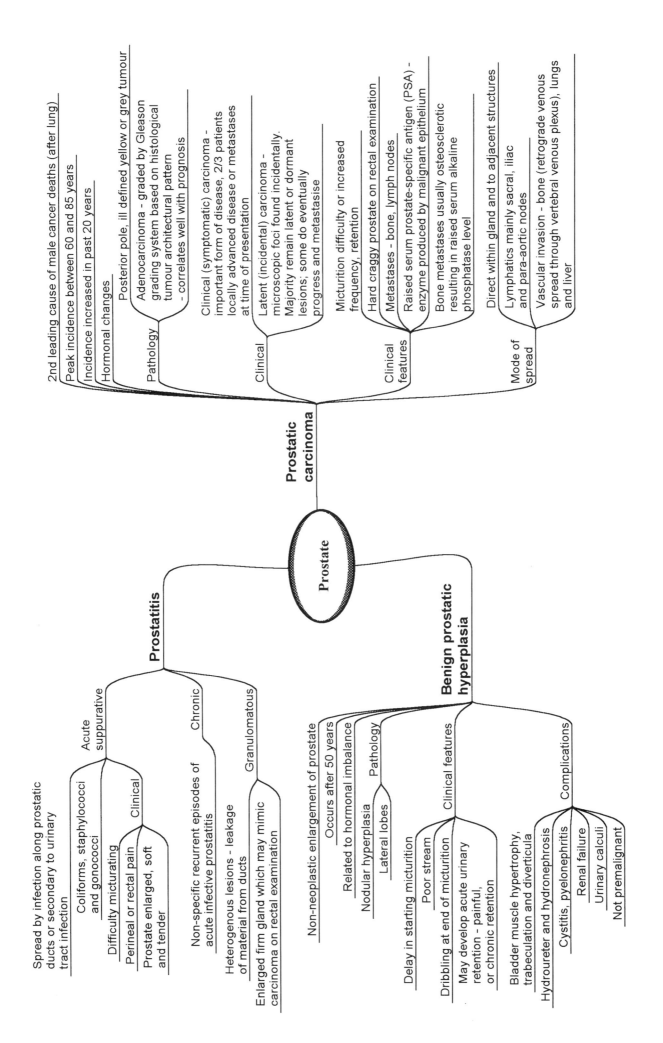

Prostate

Prostatic carcinoma

2nd leading cause of male cancer deaths (after lung)

Peak incidence between 60 and 85 years

Incidence increased in past 20 years

Hormonal changes

Pathology

Posterior pole, ill defined yellow or grey tumour

Adenocarcinoma - graded by Gleason grading system based on histological tumour architectural pattern - correlates well with prognosis

Clinical

Clinical (symptomatic) carcinoma - important form of disease, 2/3 patients locally advanced disease or metastases at time of presentation

Latent (incidental) carcinoma - microscopic foci found incidentally. Majority remain latent or dormant lesions; some do eventually progress and metastasise

Clinical features

Micturition difficulty or increased frequency, retention

Hard craggy prostate on rectal examination

Metastases - bone, lymph nodes

Raised serum prostate-specific antigen (PSA) - enzyme produced by malignant epithelium

Bone metastases usually osteosclerotic resulting in raised serum alkaline phosphatase level

Mode of spread

Direct within gland and to adjacent structures

Lymphatics mainly sacral, iliac and para-aortic nodes

Vascular invasion - bone (retrograde venous spread through vertebral venous plexus), lungs and liver

Prostatitis

Acute suppurative

Spread by infection along prostatic ducts or secondary to urinary tract infection

Coliforms, staphylococci and gonococci

Clinical

Difficulty micturating

Perineal or rectal pain

Prostate enlarged, soft and tender

Chronic

Non-specific recurrent episodes of acute infective prostatitis

Granulomatous

Heterogenous lesions - leakage of material from ducts

Enlarged firm gland which may mimic carcinoma on rectal examination

Benign prostatic hyperplasia

Non-neoplastic enlargement of prostate

Occurs after 50 years

Related to hormonal imbalance

Pathology

Nodular hyperplasia

Lateral lobes

Clinical features

Delay in starting micturition

Poor stream

Dribbling at end of micturition

May develop acute urinary retention - painful, or chronic retention

Complications

Bladder muscle hypertrophy, trabeculation and diverticula

Hydroureter and hydronephrosis

Cystitis, pyelonephritis

Renal failure

Urinary calculi

Not premalignant

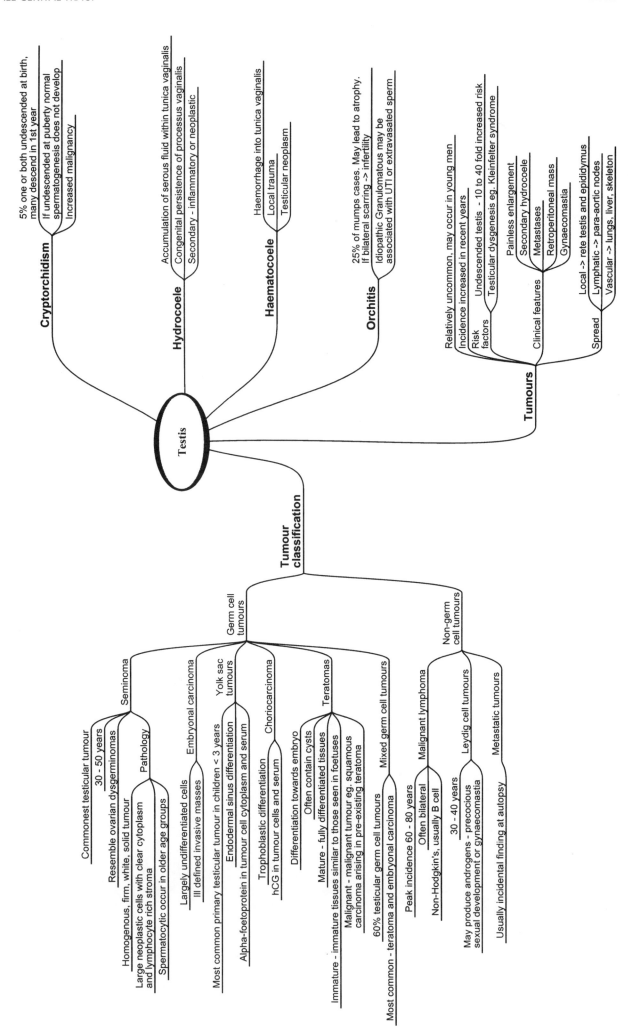

Testis

Cryptorchidism
- 5% one or both undescended at birth, many descend in 1st year
- If undescended at puberty normal spermatogenesis does not develop
- Increased malignancy

Hydrocoele
- Accumulation of serous fluid within tunica vaginalis
- Congenital persistence of processus vaginalis
- Secondary - inflammatory or neoplastic

Haematocoele
- Haemorrhage into tunica vaginalis
- Local trauma
- Testicular neoplasm

Orchitis
- 25% of mumps cases. May lead to atrophy. If bilateral scarring -> infertility
- Idiopathic Granulomatous may be associated with UTI or extravasated sperm

Tumours
- Relatively uncommon, may occur in young men
- Incidence increased in recent years
- Risk factors
  - Undescended testis - 10 to 40 fold increased risk
  - Testicular dysgenesis eg. Kleinfelter syndrome
- Clinical features
  - Painless enlargement
  - Secondary hydrocoele
  - Metastases
  - Retroperitoneal mass
  - Gynaecomastia
- Spread
  - Local -> rete testis and epididymus
  - Lymphatic -> para-aortic nodes
  - Vascular -> lungs, liver, skeleton

Tumour classification

Germ cell tumours
- Seminoma
  - Commonest testicular tumour
  - 30 - 50 years
  - Resemble ovarian dysgerminomas
  - Pathology
    - Homogenous, firm, white, solid tumour
    - Large neoplastic cells with clear cytoplasm and lymphocyte rich stroma
    - Spermatocytic occur in older age groups
- Embryonal carcinoma
  - Largely undifferentiated cells
  - Ill defined invasive masses
- Yolk sac tumours
  - Most common primary testicular tumour in children < 3 years
  - Endodermal sinus differentiation
  - Alpha-foetoprotein in tumour cell cytoplasm and serum
- Choriocarcinoma
  - Trophoblastic differentiation
  - hCG in tumour cells and serum
  - Differentiation towards embryo
- Teratomas
  - Often contain cysts
  - Mature - fully differentiated tissues
  - Immature - immature tissues similar to those seen in foetuses
  - Malignant - malignant tumour eg. squamous carcinoma arising in pre-existing teratoma
- Mixed germ cell tumours
  - 60% testicular germ cell tumours
  - Most common - teratoma and embryonal carcinoma

Non-germ cell tumours
- Malignant lymphoma
  - Peak incidence 60 - 80 years
  - Often bilateral
  - Non-Hodgkin's, usually B cell
- Leydig cell tumours
  - 30 - 40 years
  - May produce androgens - precocious sexual development or gynaecomastia
- Metastatic tumours
  - Usually incidental finding at autopsy

SYSTEMATIC PATHOLOGY

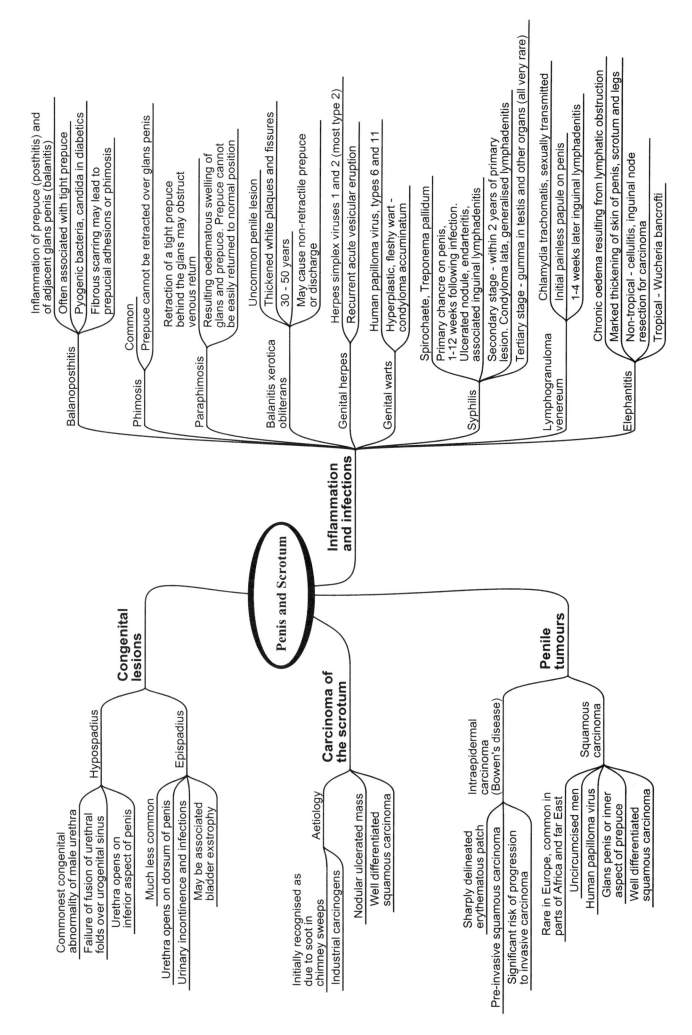

Penis and Scrotum

Inflammation and infections

Balanoposthitis
- Inflammation of prepuce (posthitis) and of adjacent glans penis (balanitis)
- Often associated with tight prepuce
- Pyogenic bacteria, candida in diabetics
- Fibrous scarring may lead to prepucial adhesions or phimosis

Phimosis
- Common
- Prepuce cannot be retracted over glans penis

Paraphimosis
- Retraction of a tight prepuce behind the glans may obstruct venous return
- Resulting oedematous swelling of glans and prepuce. Prepuce cannot be easily returned to normal position

Balanitis xerotica obliterans
- Uncommon penile lesion
- Thickened white plaques and fissures
- 30 - 50 years
- May cause non-retractile prepuce or discharge

Genital herpes
- Herpes simplex viruses 1 and 2 (most type 2)
- Recurrent acute vesicular eruption

Genital warts
- Human papilloma virus, types 6 and 11
- Hyperplastic, fleshy wart - condyloma accuminatum

Syphilis
- Spirochaete, Treponema pallidum
- Primary chancre on penis, 1-12 weeks following infection. Ulcerated nodule, endarteritis, associated inguinal lymphadenitis
- Secondary stage - within 2 years of primary lesion. Condyloma lata, generalised lymphadenitis
- Tertiary stage - gumma in testis and other organs (all very rare)

Lymphogranuloma venereum
- Chlamydia trachomatis, sexually transmitted
- Initial painless papule on penis
- 1-4 weeks later inguinal lymphadenitis

Elephantitis
- Chronic oedema resulting from lymphatic obstruction
- Marked thickening of skin of penis, scrotum and legs
- Non-tropical - cellulitis, inguinal node resection for carcinoma
- Tropical - Wucheria bancrofti

Congenital lesions

Hypospadius
- Commonest congenital abnormality of male urethra
- Failure of fusion of urethral folds over urogenital sinus
- Urethra opens on inferior aspect of penis

Epispadius
- Much less common
- Urethra opens on dorsum of penis
- Urinary incontinence and infections
- May be associated bladder exstrophy

Carcinoma of the scrotum

Aetiology
- Initially recognised as due to soot in chimney sweeps
- Industrial carcinogens

- Nodular ulcerated mass
- Well differentiated squamous carcinoma

Penile tumours

Intraepidermal carcinoma (Bowen's disease)
- Sharply delineated erythematous patch
- Pre-invasive squamous carcinoma
- Significant risk of progression to invasive carcinoma

Squamous carcinoma
- Rare in Europe, common in parts of Africa and far East
- Uncircumcised men
- Human papilloma virus
- Glans penis or inner aspect of prepuce
- Well differentiated squamous carcinoma

FEMALE GENITAL TRACT

SYSTEMATIC PATHOLOGY

SYSTEMATIC PATHOLOGY

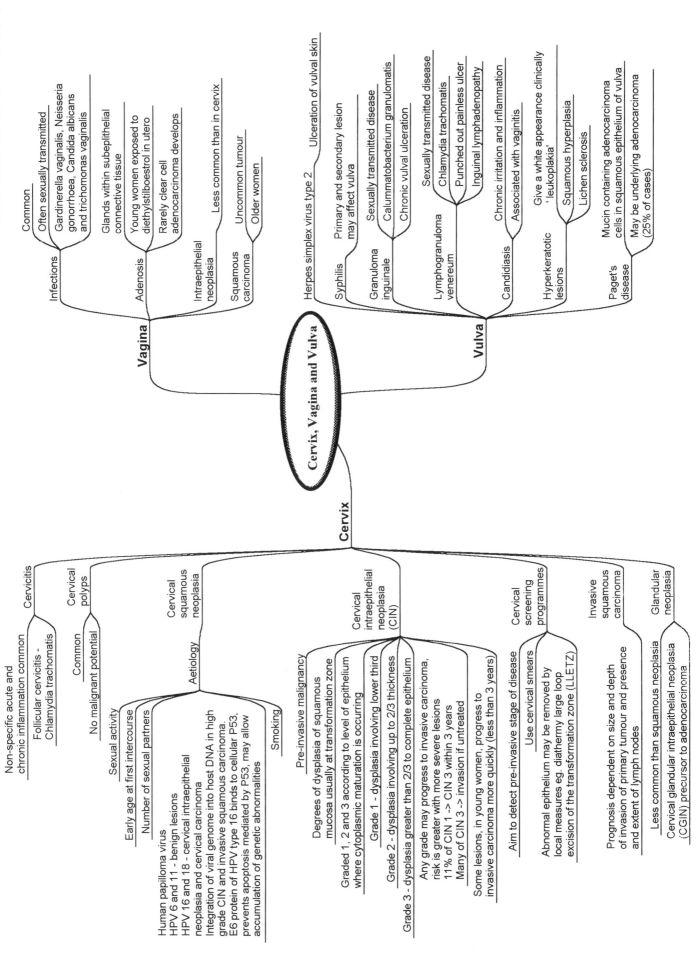

Cervix, Vagina and Vulva

Vagina

Infections
- Common
- Often sexually transmitted
- Gardinerella vaginalis, Neisseria gonorrhoea, Candida albicans and trichomonas vaginalis

Adenosis
- Glands within subepithelial connective tissue
- Young women exposed to diethylstilboestrol in utero
- Rarely clear cell adenocarcinoma develops

Intraepithelial neoplasia
- Less common than in cervix

Squamous carcinoma
- Uncommon tumour
- Older women

Vulva

Herpes simplex virus type 2
- Ulceration of vulval skin

Syphilis
- Primary and secondary lesion may affect vulva

Granuloma inguinale
- Sexually transmitted disease
- Calummatobacterium granulomatis
- Chronic vulval ulceration

Lymphogranuloma venereum
- Sexually transmitted disease
- Chlamydia trachomatis
- Punched out painless ulcer
- Inguinal lymphadenopathy

Candidiasis
- Chronic irritation and inflammation
- Associated with vaginitis

Hyperkeratotic lesions
- Give a white appearance clinically 'leukoplakia'
- Squamous hyperplasia
- Lichen sclerosis

Paget's disease
- Mucin containing adenocarcinoma cells in squamous epithelium of vulva
- May be underlying adenocarcinoma (25% of cases)

Cervix

Cervicitis
- Non-specific acute and chronic inflammation common
- Follicular cervicitis - Chlamydia trachomatis

Cervical polyps
- Common
- No malignant potential

Cervical squamous neoplasia
- Aetiology
  - Sexual activity
  - Early age at first intercourse
  - Number of sexual partners
  - Human papilloma virus
  - HPV 6 and 11 - benign lesions
  - HPV 16 and 18 - cervical intraepithelial neoplasia and cervical carcinoma
  - Integration of viral genome into host DNA in high grade CIN and invasive squamous carcinoma.
  - E6 protein of HPV type 16 binds to cellular P53, prevents apoptosis mediated by P53, may allow accumulation of genetic abnormalities
  - Smoking

Cervical intraepithelial neoplasia (CIN)
- Pre-invasive malignancy
- Degrees of dysplasia of squamous mucosa usually at transformation zone
- Graded 1, 2 and 3 according to level of epithelium where cytoplasmic maturation is occurring
- Grade 1 - dysplasia involving lower third
- Grade 2 - dysplasia involving up to 2/3 thickness
- Grade 3 - dysplasia greater than 2/3 to complete epithelium
- Any grade may progress to invasive carcinoma, risk is greater with more severe lesions
- 11% of CIN 1 -> CIN 3 within 3 years
- Many of CIN 3 -> invasion if untreated
- Some lesions, in young women, progress to invasive carcinoma more quickly (less than 3 years)

Cervical screening programmes
- Aim to detect pre-invasive stage of disease
- Use cervical smears
- Abnormal epithelium may be removed by local measures eg. diathermy large loop excision of the transformation zone (LLETZ)

Invasive squamous carcinoma
- Prognosis dependent on size and depth of invasion of primary tumour and presence and extent of lymph nodes

Glandular neoplasia
- Less common than squamous neoplasia
- Cervical glandular intraepithelial neoplasia (CGIN) precursor to adenocarcinoma

SYSTEMATIC PATHOLOGY

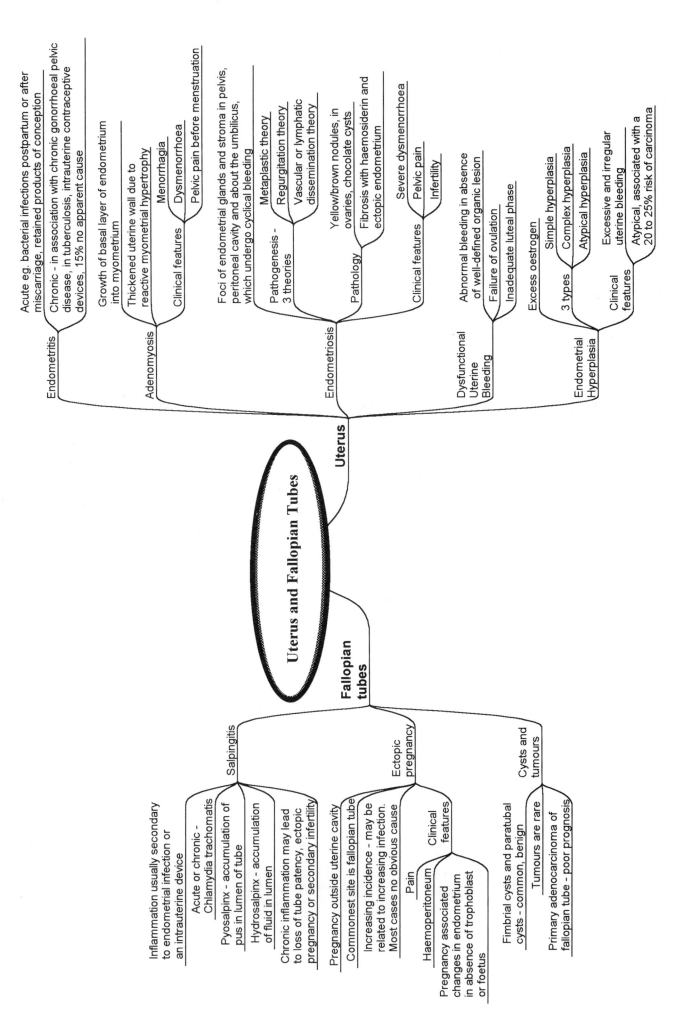

Uterus and Fallopian Tubes

Uterus

Endometritis
- Acute eg. bacterial infections postpartum or after miscarriage, retained products of conception
- Chronic - in association with chronic gonorrhoeal pelvic disease, in tuberculosis, intrauterine contraceptive devices, 15% no apparent cause

Adenomyosis
- Growth of basal layer of endometrium into myometrium
- Thickened uterine wall due to reactive myometrial hypertrophy
- Clinical features
  - Menorrhagia
  - Dysmenorrhoea
  - Pelvic pain before menstruation

Endometriosis
- Foci of endometrial glands and stroma in pelvis, peritoneal cavity and about the umbilicus, which undergo cyclical bleeding
- Pathogenesis - 3 theories
  - Metaplastic theory
  - Regurgitation theory
  - Vascular or lymphatic dissemination theory
- Pathology
  - Yellow/brown nodules, in ovaries, chocolate cysts
  - Fibrosis with haemosiderin and ectopic endometrium
- Clinical features
  - Severe dysmenorrhoea
  - Pelvic pain
  - Infertility

Dysfunctional Uterine Bleeding
- Abnormal bleeding in absence of well-defined organic lesion
- Failure of ovulation
- Inadequate luteal phase

Endometrial Hyperplasia
- Excess oestrogen
- 3 types
  - Simple hyperplasia
  - Complex hyperplasia
  - Atypical hyperplasia
- Clinical features
  - Excessive and irregular uterine bleeding
  - Atypical, associated with a 20 to 25% risk of carcinoma

Fallopian tubes

Salpingitis
- Inflammation usually secondary to endometrial infection or an intrauterine device
- Acute or chronic - Chlamydia trachomatis
- Pyosalpinx - accumulation of pus in lumen of tube
- Hydrosalpinx - accumulation of fluid in lumen
- Chronic inflammation may lead to loss of tube patency, ectopic pregnancy or secondary infertility

Ectopic pregnancy
- Pregnancy outside uterine cavity
- Commonest site is fallopian tube
- Increasing incidence - may be related to increasing infection. Most cases no obvious cause
- Clinical features
  - Pain
  - Haemoperitoneum
  - Pregnancy associated changes in endometrium in absence of trophoblast or foetus

Cysts and tumours
- Fimbrial cysts and paratubal cysts - common, benign
- Tumours are rare
- Primary adenocarcinoma of fallopian tube - poor prognosis

SYSTEMATIC PATHOLOGY

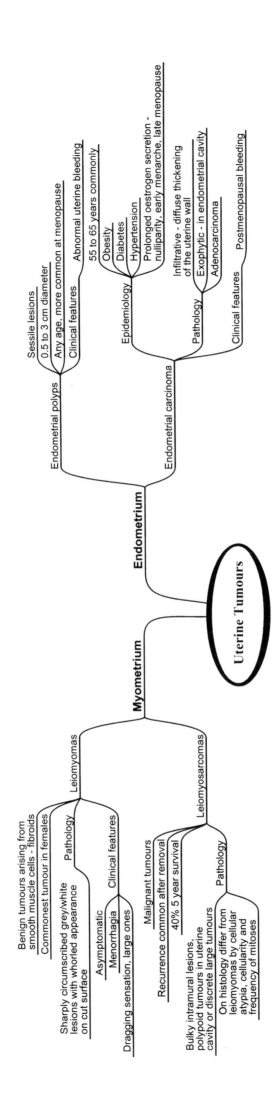

Uterine Tumours

Endometrium

Endometrial polyps
- Sessile lesions
- 0.5 to 3 cm diameter
- Any age, more common at menopause
- Clinical features
  - Abnormal uterine bleeding

Endometrial carcinoma
- Epidemiology
  - 55 to 65 years commonly
  - Obesity
  - Diabetes
  - Hypertension
  - Prolonged oestrogen secretion - nulliparity, early menarche, late menopause
- Pathology
  - Infiltrative - diffuse thickening of the uterine wall
  - Exophytic - in endometrial cavity
  - Adenocarcinoma
- Clinical features
  - Postmenopausal bleeding

Myometrium

Leiomyomas
- Benign tumours arising from smooth muscle cells - fibroids
- Commonest tumour in females
- Pathology
  - Sharply circumscribed grey/white lesions with whorled appearance on cut surface
- Clinical features
  - Asymptomatic
  - Menorrhagia
  - Dragging sensation, large ones

Leiomyosarcomas
- Malignant tumours
- Recurrence common after removal
- 40% 5 year survival
- Pathology
  - Bulky intramural lesions, polypoid tumours in uterine cavity or discrete large tumours
  - On histology differ from leiomyomas by cellular atypia, cellularity and frequency of mitoses

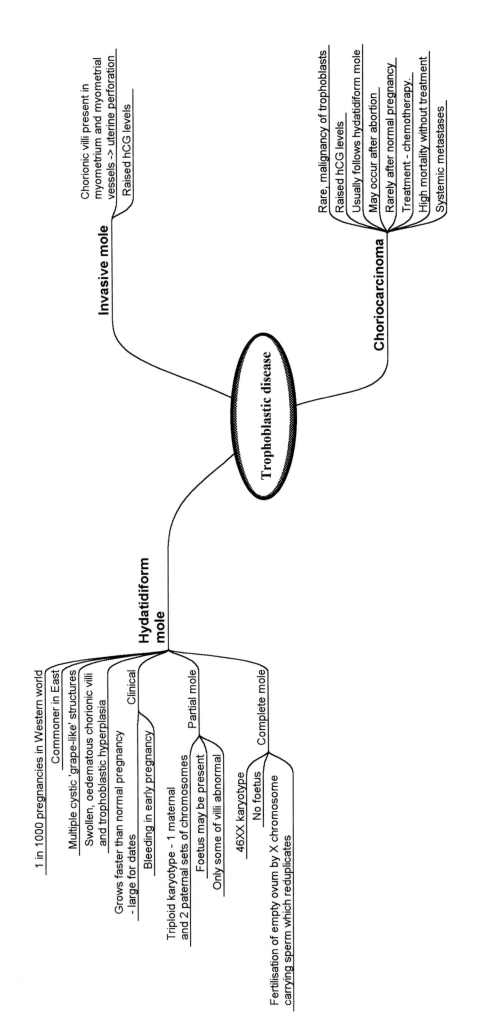

Trophoblastic disease

Invasive mole
- Chorionic villi present in myometrium and myometrial vessels -> uterine perforation
- Raised hCG levels

Choriocarcinoma
- Rare, malignancy of trophoblasts
- Raised hCG levels
- Usually follows hydatidiform mole
- May occur after abortion
- Rarely after normal pregnancy
- Treatment - chemotherapy.
- High mortality without treatment
- Systemic metastases

Hydatidiform mole
- 1 in 1000 pregnancies in Western world
- Commoner in East
- Multiple cystic 'grape-like' structures
- Swollen, oedematous chorionic villi and trophoblastic hyperplasia

Clinical
- Grows faster than normal pregnancy - large for dates
- Bleeding in early pregnancy

Partial mole
- Triploid karyotype - 1 maternal and 2 paternal sets of chromosomes
- Foetus may be present
- Only some of villi abnormal

Complete mole
- 46XX karyotype
- No foetus
- Fertilisation of empty ovum by X chromosome carrying sperm which reduplicates

SYSTEMATIC PATHOLOGY

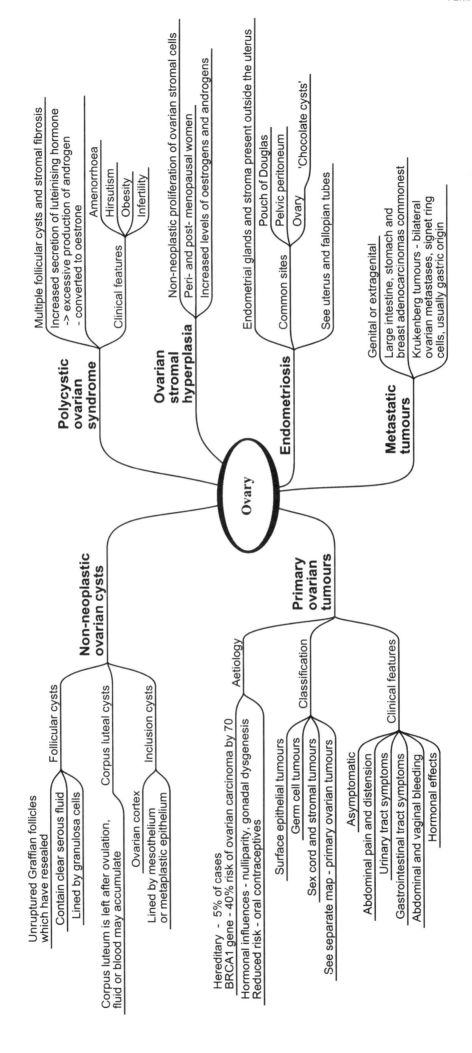

Ovary

Polycystic ovarian syndrome

Multiple follicular cysts and stromal fibrosis

Increased secretion of luteinising hormone
-> excessive production of androgen
- converted to oestrone

Clinical features
- Amenorrhoea
- Hirsutism
- Obesity
- Infertility

Ovarian stromal hyperplasia

Non-neoplastic proliferation of ovarian stromal cells

Peri- and post- menopausal women

Increased levels of oestrogens and androgens

Endometriosis

Endometrial glands and stroma present outside the uterus

Common sites
- Pouch of Douglas
- Pelvic peritoneum
- Ovary — 'Chocolate cysts'

See uterus and fallopian tubes

Metastatic tumours

Genital or extragenital

Large intestine, stomach and breast adenocarcinomas commonest

Krukenberg tumours - bilateral ovarian metastases, signet ring cells, usually gastric origin

Non-neoplastic ovarian cysts

Follicular cysts
- Unruptured Graffian follicles which have resealed
- Contain clear serous fluid
- Lined by granulosa cells

Corpus luteal cysts
- Corpus luteum is left after ovulation, fluid or blood may accumulate

Inclusion cysts
- Ovarian cortex
- Lined by mesothelium or metaplastic epithelium

Primary ovarian tumours

Aetiology
- Hereditary - 5% of cases
- BRCA1 gene - 40% risk of ovarian carcinoma by 70
- Hormonal influences - nulliparity, gonadal dysgenesis
- Reduced risk - oral contraceptives

Classification
- Surface epithelial tumours
- Germ cell tumours
- Sex cord and stromal tumours
- See separate map - primary ovarian tumours

Clinical features
- Asymptomatic
- Abdominal pain and distension
- Urinary tract symptoms
- Gastrointestinal tract symptoms
- Abdominal and vaginal bleeding
- Hormonal effects

SYSTEMATIC PATHOLOGY

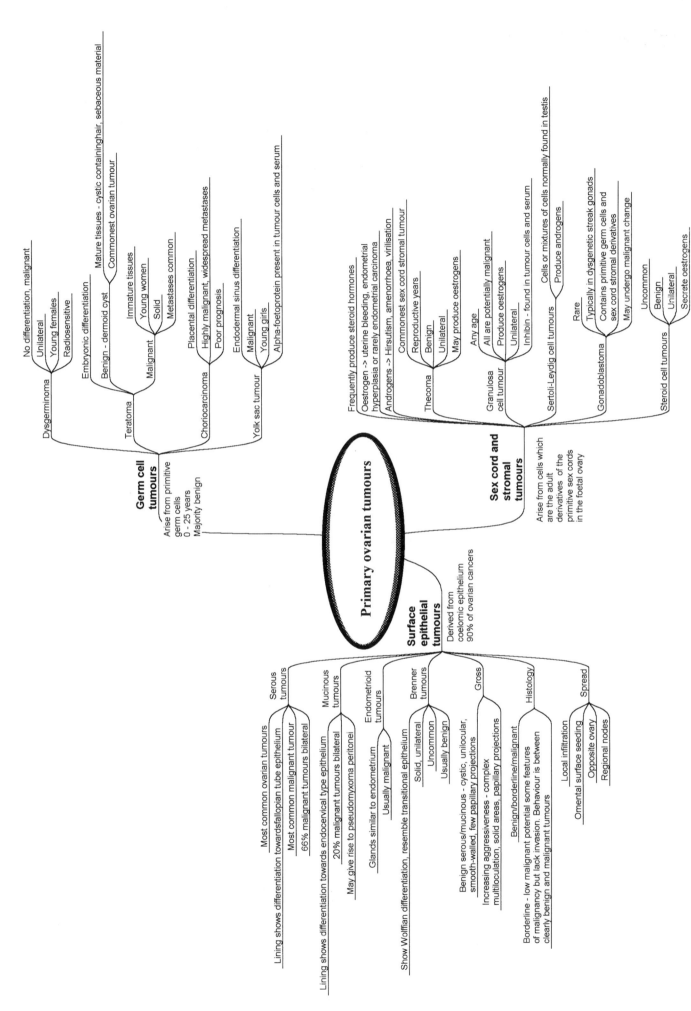

Primary ovarian tumours

Germ cell tumours
Arise from primitive germ cells
0 - 25 years
Majority benign

Dysgerminoma
- No differentiation, malignant
- Unilateral
- Young females
- Radiosensitive

Teratoma
- Embryonic differentiation
- Benign - dermoid cyst
  - Mature tissues - cystic containing hair, sebaceous material
  - Commonest ovarian tumour
- Malignant
  - Immature tissues
  - Young women
  - Solid
  - Metastases common

Choriocarcinoma
- Placental differentiation
- Highly malignant, widespread metastases
- Poor prognosis

Yolk sac tumour
- Endodermal sinus differentiation
- Malignant
- Young girls
- Alpha-foetoprotein present in tumour cells and serum

Sex cord and stromal tumours
Arise from cells which are the adult derivatives of the primitive sex cords in the foetal ovary

- Frequently produce steroid hormones
- Oestrogen -> uterine bleeding, endometrial hyperplasia or rarely endometrial carcinoma
- Androgens -> Hirsutism, amenorrhoea, virilisation

Thecoma
- Commonest sex cord stromal tumour
- Reproductive years
- Benign
- Unilateral
- May produce oestrogens

Granulosa cell tumour
- Any age
- All are potentially malignant
- Produce oestrogens
- Unilateral
- Inhibin - found in tumour cells and serum

Sertoli-Leydig cell tumours
- Cells or mixtures of cells normally found in testis
- Produce androgens
- Rare

Gonadoblastoma
- Typically in dysgenetic streak gonads
- Contains primitive germ cells and sex cord stromal derivatives
- May undergo malignant change

Steroid cell tumours
- Uncommon
- Benign
- Unilateral
- Secrete oestrogens

Surface epithelial tumours
Derived from coelomic epithelium
90% of ovarian cancers

Serous tumours
- Most common ovarian tumours
- Lining shows differentiation towards fallopian tube epithelium
- Most common malignant tumour
- 66% malignant tumours bilateral

Mucinous tumours
- Lining shows differentiation towards endocervical type epithelium
- 20% malignant tumours bilateral
- May give rise to pseudomyxoma peritonei

Endometrioid tumours
- Glands similar to endometrium
- Usually malignant

Brenner tumours
- Show Wolffian differentiation, resemble transitional epithelium
- Solid, unilateral
- Uncommon
- Usually benign

Gross
- Benign serous/mucinous - cystic, unilocular, smooth-walled, few papillary projections
- Increasing aggressiveness - complex multiloculation, solid areas, papillary projections

Histology
- Benign/borderline/malignant
- Borderline - low malignant potential some features of malignancy but lack invasion. Behaviour is between clearly benign and malignant tumours

Spread
- Local infiltration
- Omental surface seeding
- Opposite ovary
- Regional nodes

BREAST

SYSTEMATIC PATHOLOGY

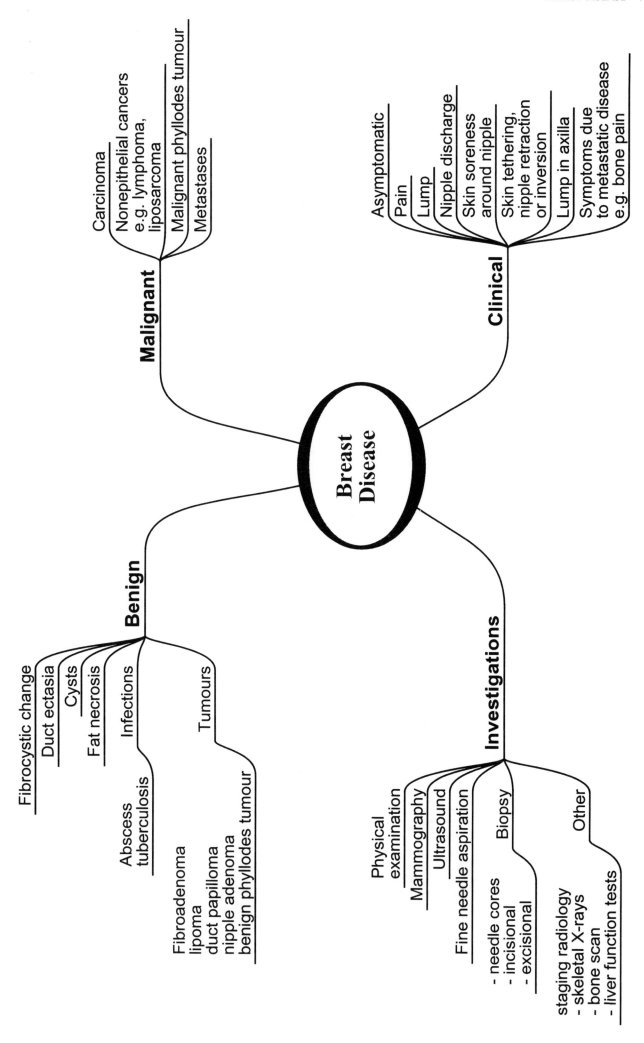

Breast Disease

Malignant
- Carcinoma
- Nonepithelial cancers e.g. lymphoma, liposarcoma
- Malignant phyllodes tumour
- Metastases

Benign
- Fibrocystic change
- Duct ectasia
- Cysts
- Fat necrosis
- Infections
  - Abscess
  - tuberculosis
- Tumours
  - Fibroadenoma
  - lipoma
  - duct papilloma
  - nipple adenoma
  - benign phyllodes tumour

Clinical
- Asymptomatic
- Pain
- Lump
- Nipple discharge
- Skin soreness around nipple
- Skin tethering, nipple retraction or inversion
- Lump in axilla
- Symptoms due to metastatic disease e.g. bone pain

Investigations
- Physical examination
- Mammography
- Ultrasound
- Fine needle aspiration
- Biopsy
  - needle cores
  - incisional
  - excisional
- Other
  - staging radiology
  - skeletal X-rays
  - bone scan
  - liver function tests

SYSTEMATIC PATHOLOGY

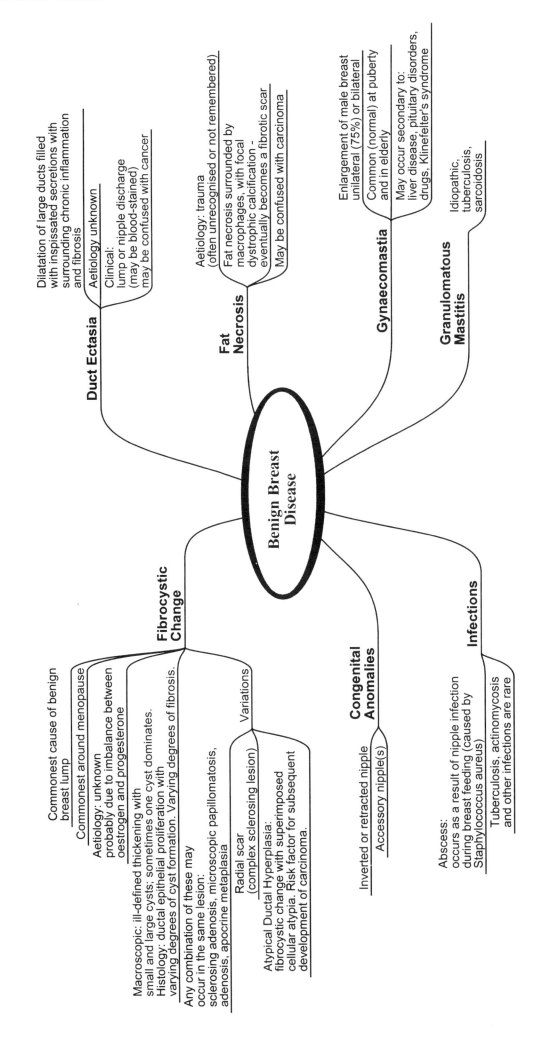

Benign Breast Disease

Duct Ectasia

Dilatation of large ducts filled with inspissated secretions with surrounding chronic inflammation and fibrosis

Aetiology: unknown

Clinical:
lump or nipple discharge
(may be blood-stained)
may be confused with cancer

Fat Necrosis

Aetiology: trauma
(often unrecognised or not remembered)

Fat necrosis surrounded by macrophages, with focal dystrophic calcification - eventually becomes a fibrotic scar

May be confused with carcinoma

Gynaecomastia

Enlargement of male breast unilateral (75%) or bilateral

Common (normal) at puberty and in elderly

May occur secondary to:
liver disease, pituitary disorders, drugs, Klinefelter's syndrome

Granulomatous Mastitis

Idiopathic, tuberculosis, sarcoidosis

Fibrocystic Change

Commonest cause of benign breast lump

Commonest around menopause

Aetiology: unknown probably due to imbalance between oestrogen and progesterone

Macroscopic: ill-defined thickening with small and large cysts; sometimes one cyst dominates. Histology: ductal epithelial proliferation with varying degrees of cyst formation. Varying degrees of fibrosis.

Variations

Any combination of these may occur in the same lesion:
sclerosing adenosis, microscopic papillomatosis, adenosis, apocrine metaplasia

Radial scar
(complex sclerosing lesion)

Atypical Ductal Hyperplasia:
fibrocystic change with superimposed cellular atypia. Risk factor for subsequent development of carcinoma.

Congenital Anomalies

Inverted or retracted nipple

Accessory nipple(s)

Infections

Abscess:
occurs as a result of nipple infection during breast feeding (caused by Staphylococcus aureus)

Tuberculosis, actinomycosis and other infections are rare

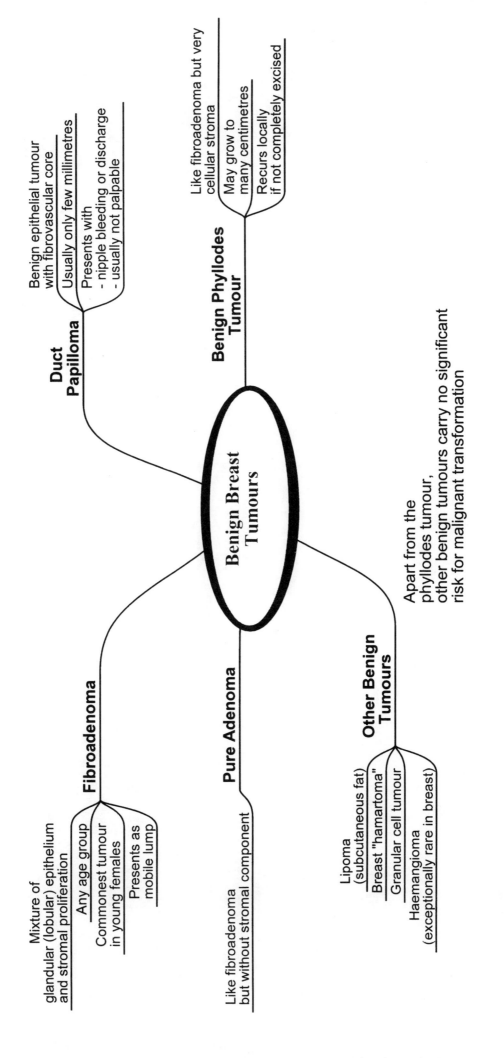

Benign Breast Tumours

Duct Papilloma

Benign epithelial tumour with fibrovascular core

Usually only few millimetres

Presents with
- nipple bleeding or discharge
- usually not palpable

Benign Phyllodes Tumour

Like fibroadenoma but very cellular stroma

May grow to many centimetres

Recurs locally if not completely excised

Fibroadenoma

Mixture of glandular (lobular) epithelium and stromal proliferation

Any age group

Commonest tumour in young females

Presents as mobile lump

Pure Adenoma

Like fibroadenoma but without stromal component

Other Benign Tumours

Apart from the phyllodes tumour, other benign tumours carry no significant risk for malignant transformation

Lipoma (subcutaneous fat)

Breast "hamartoma"

Granular cell tumour

Haemangioma (exceptionally rare in breast)

SYSTEMATIC PATHOLOGY

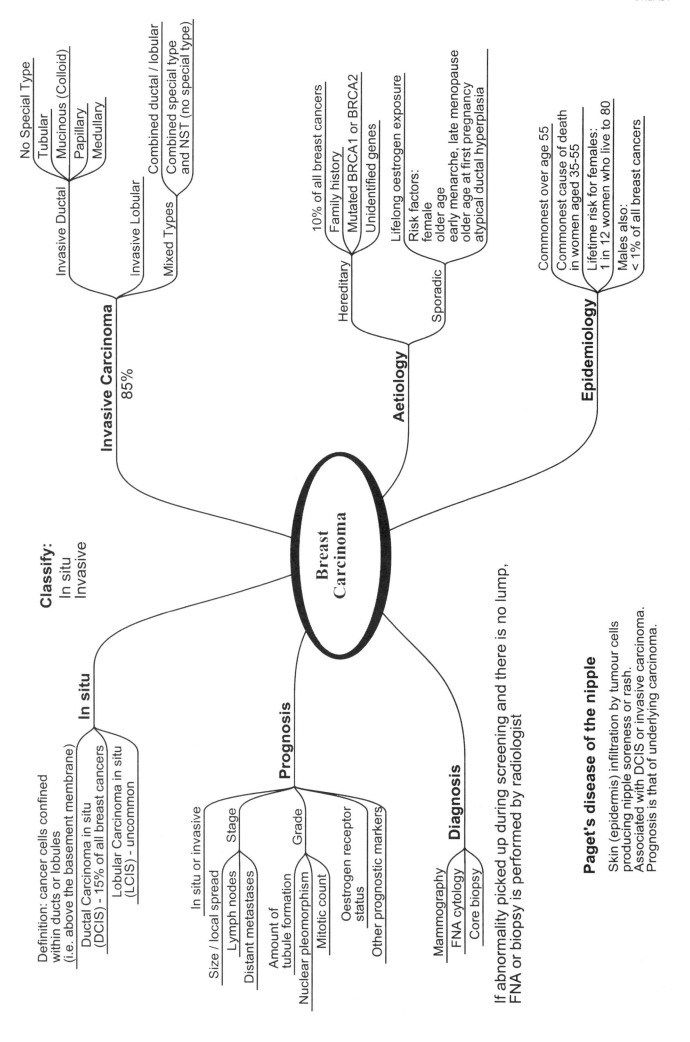

Breast Carcinoma

Invasive Carcinoma 85%

Invasive Ductal
- No Special Type
  - Tubular
  - Mucinous (Colloid)
  - Papillary
  - Medullary

Invasive Lobular

Mixed Types
- Combined ductal / lobular
- Combined special type and NST (no special type)

Classify:
In situ
Invasive

In situ

Definition: cancer cells confined within ducts or lobules (i.e. above the basement membrane)

Ductal Carcinoma in situ (DCIS) - 15% of all breast cancers

Lobular Carcinoma in situ (LCIS) - uncommon

Aetiology

Hereditary
- 10% of all breast cancers
- Family history
- Mutated BRCA1 or BRCA2
- Unidentified genes

Sporadic
- Lifelong oestrogen exposure
- Risk factors:
  female
  older age
  early menarche, late menopause
  older age at first pregnancy
  atypical ductal hyperplasia

Epidemiology
- Commonest over age 55
- Commonest cause of death in women aged 35-55
- Lifetime risk for females: 1 in 12 women who live to 80
- Males also: < 1% of all breast cancers

Prognosis
- In situ or invasive
- Size / local spread
- Stage
  - Lymph nodes
  - Distant metastases
- Grade
  - Amount of tubule formation
  - Nuclear pleomorphism
  - Mitotic count
- Oestrogen receptor status
- Other prognostic markers

Diagnosis
- Mammography
- FNA cytology
- Core biopsy

If abnormality picked up during screening and there is no lump, FNA or biopsy is performed by radiologist

Paget's disease of the nipple

Skin (epidermis) infiltration by tumour cells producing nipple soreness or rash.
Associated with DCIS or invasive carcinoma.
Prognosis is that of underlying carcinoma.

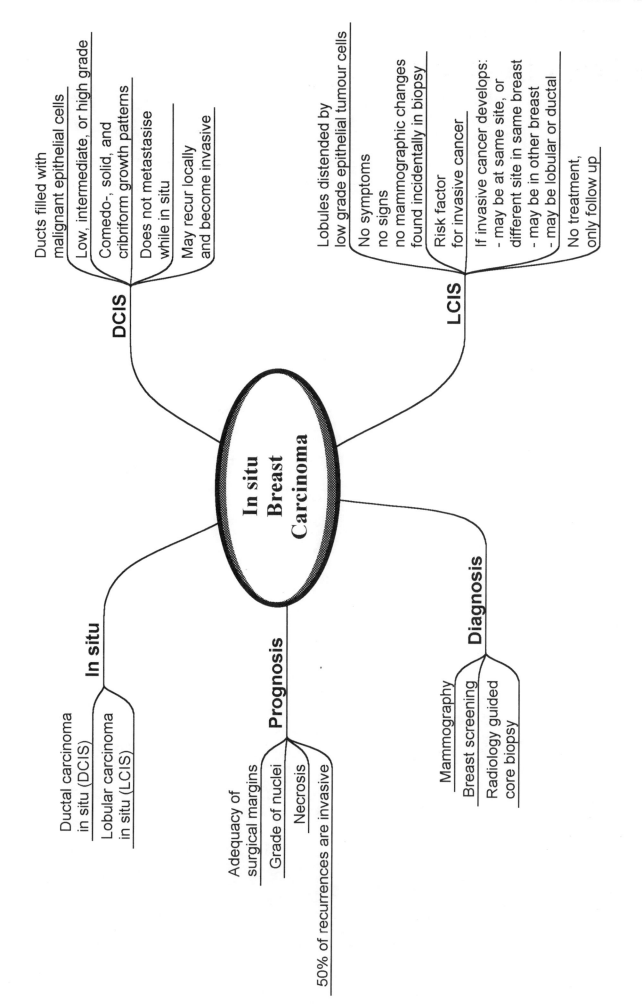

In situ Breast Carcinoma

DCIS
- Ducts filled with malignant epithelial cells
- Low, intermediate, or high grade
- Comedo-, solid, and cribriform growth patterns
- Does not metastasise while in situ
- May recur locally and become invasive

LCIS
- Lobules distended by low grade epithelial tumour cells
- No symptoms no signs no mammographic changes found incidentally in biopsy
- Risk factor for invasive cancer
- If invasive cancer develops:
  - may be at same site, or different site in same breast
  - may be in other breast
  - may be lobular or ductal
- No treatment, only follow up

In situ
- Ductal carcinoma in situ (DCIS)
- Lobular carcinoma in situ (LCIS)

Prognosis
- Adequacy of surgical margins
- Grade of nuclei
- Necrosis
- 50% of recurrences are invasive

Diagnosis
- Mammography
- Breast screening
- Radiology guided core biopsy

BLOOD AND
BONE MARROW

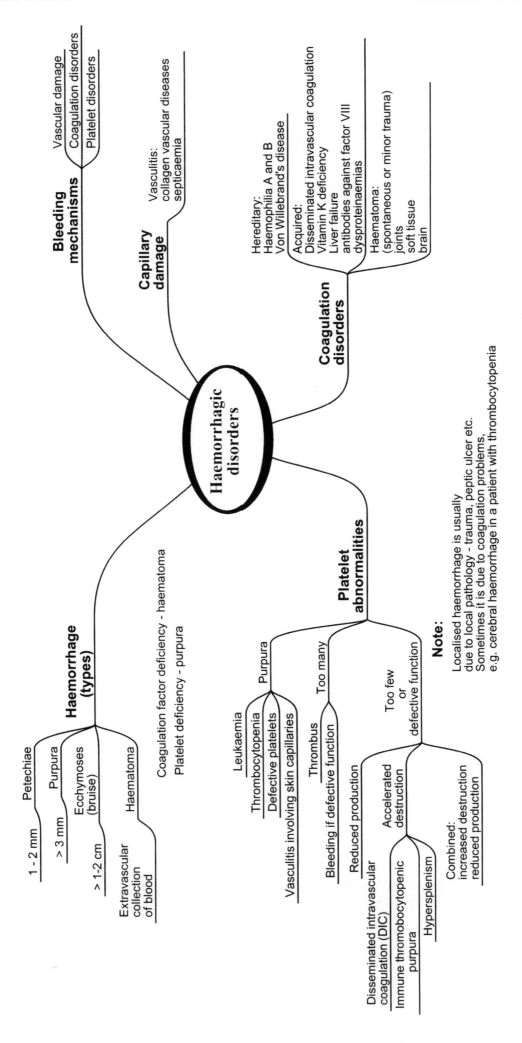

Haemorrhagic disorders

Bleeding mechanisms
- Vascular damage
- Coagulation disorders
- Platelet disorders

Capillary damage
- Vasculitis:
  - collagen vascular diseases
  - septicaemia

Coagulation disorders
- Hereditary:
  - Haemophilia A and B
  - Von Willebrand's disease
- Acquired:
  - Disseminated intravascular coagulation
  - Vitamin K deficiency
  - Liver failure
  - antibodies against factor VIII
  - dysproteinaemias
- Haematoma: (spontaneous or minor trauma)
  - joints
  - soft tissue
  - brain

Haemorrhage (types)
- Petechiae — 1 - 2 mm
- Purpura — > 3 mm
- Ecchymoses (bruise) — > 1-2 cm
- Haematoma — Extravascular collection of blood
- Coagulation factor deficiency - haematoma
- Platelet deficiency - purpura

Platelet abnormalities
- Purpura
  - Leukaemia
  - Thrombocytopenia
  - Defective platelets
  - Vasculitis involving skin capillaries
- Too many
  - Thrombus
  - Bleeding if defective function
- Too few or defective function
  - Reduced production
  - Accelerated destruction
    - Disseminated intravascular coagulation (DIC)
    - Immune thrombocytopenic purpura
    - Hypersplenism
  - Combined: increased destruction reduced production

Note:
Localised haemorrhage is usually due to local pathology - trauma, peptic ulcer etc. Sometimes it is due to coagulation problems, e.g. cerebral haemorrhage in a patient with thrombocytopenia

SYSTEMATIC PATHOLOGY

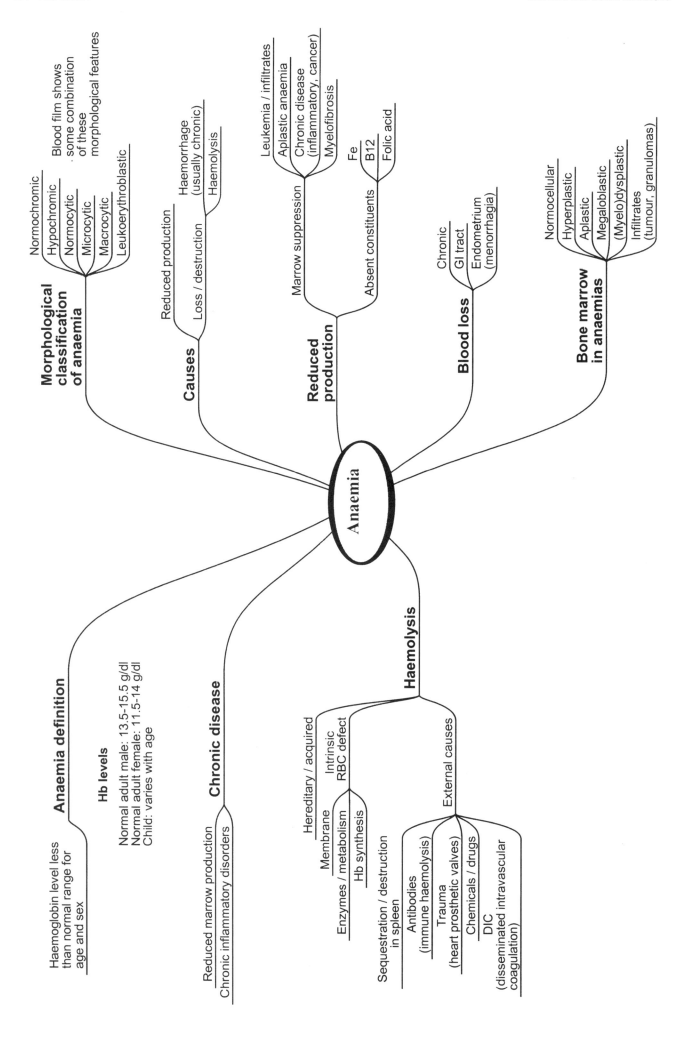

Morphological classification of anaemia

- Normochromic
- Hypochromic
- Normocytic
- Microcytic
- Macrocytic
- Leukoerythroblastic

Blood film shows some combination of these morphological features

Causes

- Reduced production
- Loss / destruction
  - Haemorrhage (usually chronic)
  - Haemolysis

Reduced production

- Marrow suppression
  - Leukemia / infiltrates
  - Aplastic anaemia
  - Chronic disease (inflammatory, cancer)
  - Myelofibrosis
- Absent constituents
  - Fe
  - B12
  - Folic acid

Blood loss

- Chronic
- GI tract
- Endometrium (menorrhagia)

Bone marrow in anaemias

- Normocellular
- Hyperplastic
- Aplastic
- Megaloblastic
- (Myelo)dysplastic
- Infiltrates (tumour, granulomas)

Anaemia

Anaemia definition

Haemoglobin level less than normal range for age and sex

Hb levels

Normal adult male: 13.5-15.5 g/dl
Normal adult female: 11.5-14 g/dl
Child: varies with age

Chronic disease

- Reduced marrow production
- Chronic inflammatory disorders

Haemolysis

- Hereditary / acquired
  - Intrinsic RBC defect
    - Membrane
    - Enzymes / metabolism
    - Hb synthesis
- External causes
  - Sequestration / destruction in spleen
  - Antibodies (immune haemolysis)
  - Trauma (heart prosthetic valves)
  - Chemicals / drugs
  - DIC (disseminated intravascular coagulation)

SYSTEMATIC PATHOLOGY

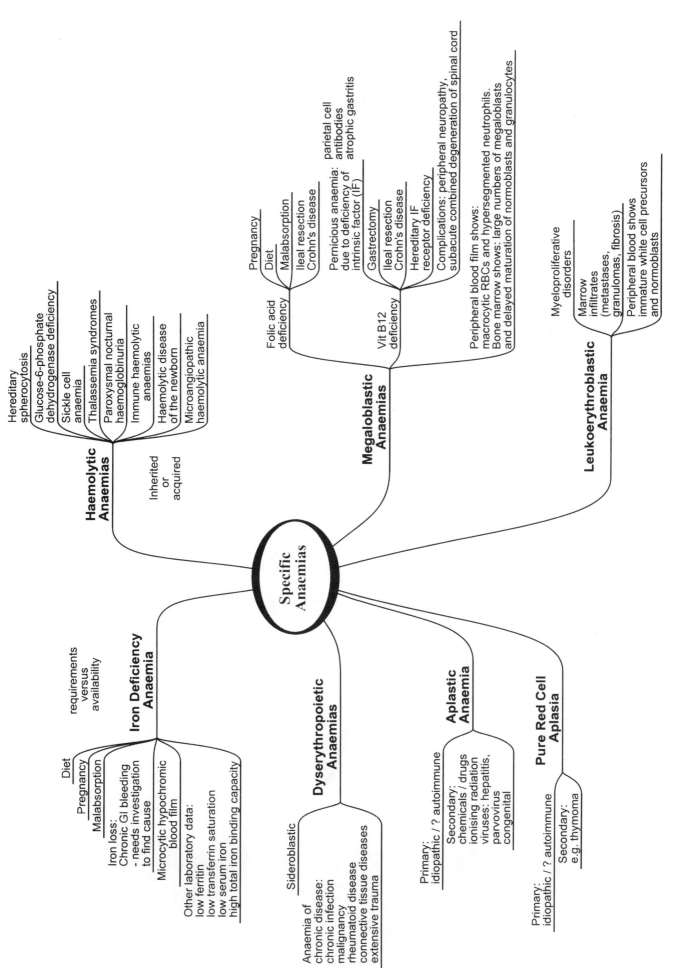

Specific Anaemias

Haemolytic Anaemias

Inherited or acquired

- Hereditary spherocytosis
- Glucose-6-phosphate dehydrogenase deficiency
- Sickle cell anaemia
- Thalassemia syndromes
- Paroxysmal nocturnal haemoglobinuria
- Immune haemolytic anaemias
- Haemolytic disease of the newborn
- Microangiopathic haemolytic anaemia

Megaloblastic Anaemias

Folic acid deficiency
- Pregnancy
- Diet
- Malabsorption
- Ileal resection Crohn's disease

Vit B12 deficiency
- Pernicious anaemia: due to deficiency of intrinsic factor (IF)
  - parietal cell antibodies atrophic gastritis
- Gastrectomy
- Ileal resection Crohn's disease
- Hereditary IF receptor deficiency
- Complications: peripheral neuropathy, subacute combined degeneration of spinal cord

Peripheral blood film shows: macrocytic RBCs and hypersegmented neutrophils. Bone marrow shows: large numbers of megaloblasts and delayed maturation of normoblasts and granulocytes

Leukoerythroblastic Anaemia

- Myeloproliferative disorders
- Marrow infiltrates (metastases, granulomas, fibrosis)
- Peripheral blood shows immature white cell precursors and normoblasts

Iron Deficiency Anaemia

requirements versus availability

- Diet
- Pregnancy
- Malabsorption
- Iron loss: Chronic GI bleeding – needs investigation to find cause
- Microcytic hypochromic blood film
- Other laboratory data: low ferritin low transferrin saturation low serum iron high total iron binding capacity

Dyserythropoietic Anaemias

- Sideroblastic
- Anaemia of chronic disease: chronic infection malignancy rheumatoid disease connective tissue diseases extensive trauma

Aplastic Anaemia

- Primary: idiopathic / ? autoimmune
- Secondary: chemicals / drugs ionising radiation viruses: hepatitis, parvovirus congenital

Pure Red Cell Aplasia

- Primary: idiopathic / ? autoimmune
- Secondary: e.g. thymoma

SYSTEMATIC PATHOLOGY

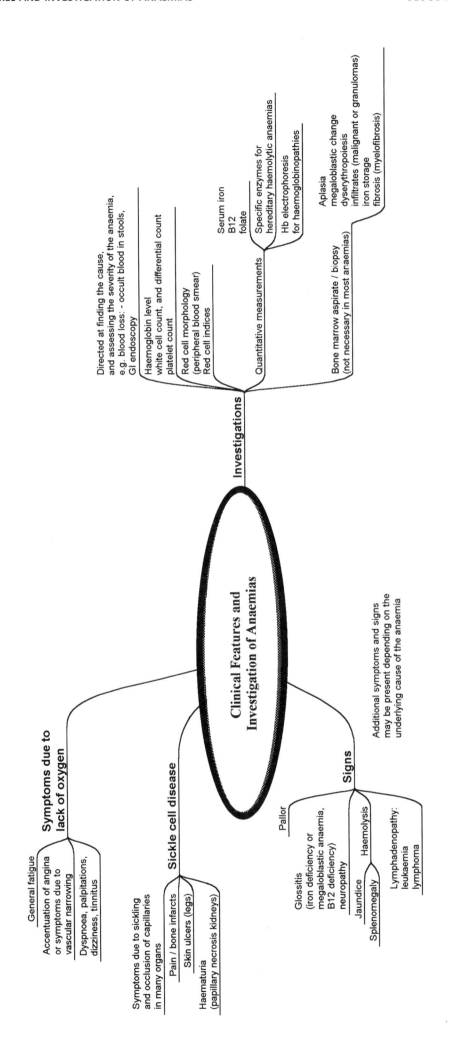

Clinical Features and Investigation of Anaemias

Investigations

Directed at finding the cause, and assessing the severity of the anaemia, e.g. blood loss: - occult blood in stools, GI endoscopy

Haemoglobin level
white cell count, and differential count
platelet count

Red cell morphology
(peripheral blood smear)
Red cell indices

Quantitative measurements

Serum iron
B12
folate

Specific enzymes for hereditary haemolytic anaemias

Hb electrophoresis for haemoglobinopathies

Bone marrow aspirate / biopsy
(not necessary in most anaemias)

Aplasia
megaloblastic change
dyserythropoiesis
infiltrates (malignant or granulomas)
iron storage
fibrosis (myelofibrosis)

Symptoms due to lack of oxygen

General fatigue
Accentuation of angina or symptoms due to vascular narrowing
Dyspnoea, palpitations, dizziness, tinnitus

Sickle cell disease

Symptoms due to sickling and occlusion of capillaries in many organs

Pain / bone infarcts
Skin ulcers (legs)
Haematuria
(papillary necrosis kidneys)

Signs

Additional symptoms and signs may be present depending on the underlying cause of the anaemia

Pallor
Glossitis
(iron deficiency or megaloblastic anaemia, B12 deficiency)
neuropathy
Jaundice — Haemolysis
Splenomegaly
Lymphadenopathy:
leukaemia
lymphoma

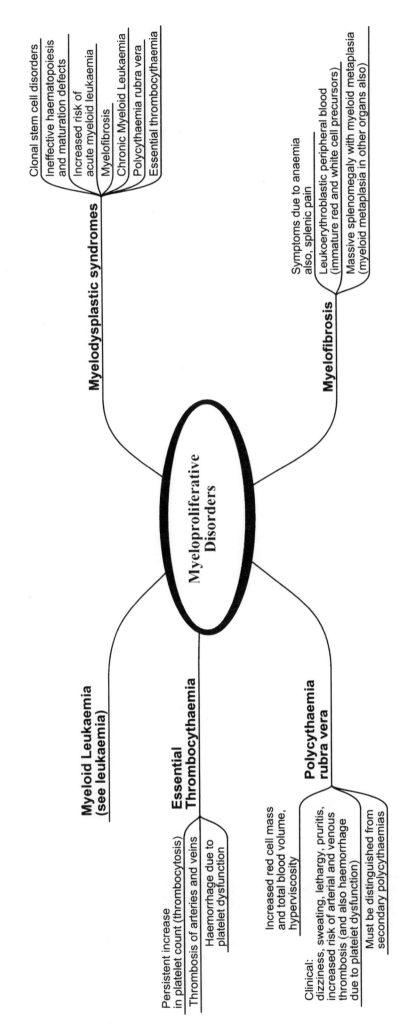

Myeloproliferative Disorders

Myelodysplastic syndromes

- Clonal stem cell disorders
- Ineffective haematopoiesis and maturation defects
- Increased risk of acute myeloid leukaemia
- Myelofibrosis
- Chronic Myeloid Leukaemia
- Polycythaemia rubra vera
- Essential thrombocythaemia

Myelofibrosis

- Symptoms due to anaemia also, splenic pain
- Leukoerythroblastic peripheral blood (immature red and white cell precursors)
- Massive splenomegaly with myeloid metaplasia (myeloid metaplasia in other organs also)

Myeloid Leukaemia (see leukaemia)

Essential Thrombocythaemia

- Persistent increase in platelet count (thrombocytosis)
- Thrombosis of arteries and veins
- Haemorrhage due to platelet dysfunction

Polycythaemia rubra vera

- Increased red cell mass and total blood volume, hyperviscosity
- Clinical: dizziness, sweating, lethargy, pruritis, increased risk of arterial and venous thrombosis (and also haemorrhage due to platelet dysfunction)
- Must be distinguished from secondary polycythaemias

LEUKAEMIAS AND LYMPHOMAS

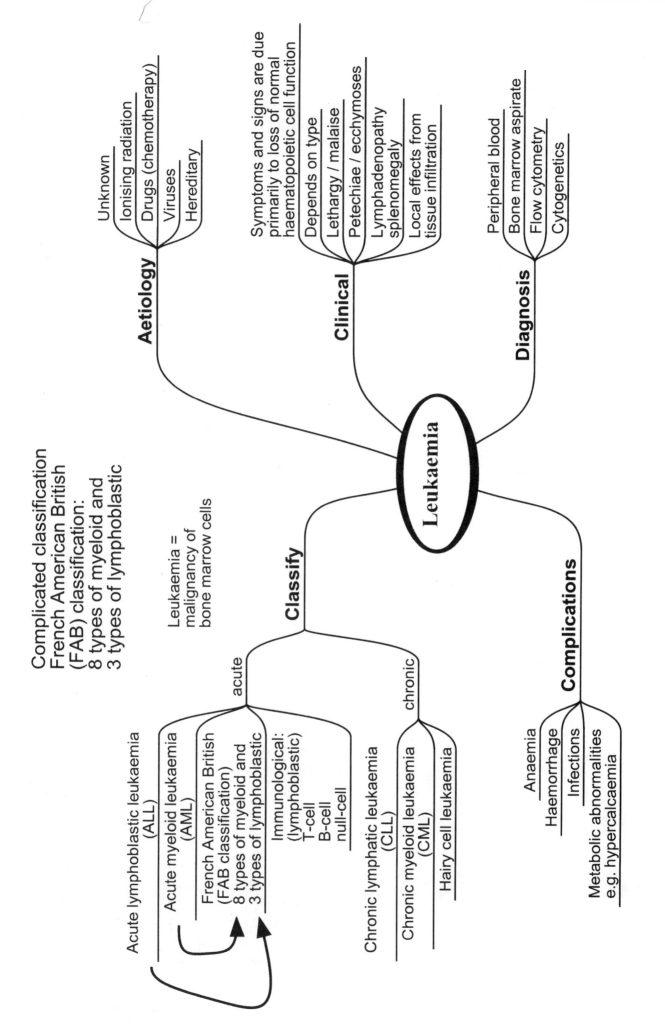

Leukaemia

Aetiology
- Unknown
- Ionising radiation
- Drugs (chemotherapy)
- Viruses
- Hereditary

Clinical
- Symptoms and signs are due primarily to loss of normal haematopoietic cell function
- Depends on type
- Lethargy / malaise
- Petechiae / ecchymoses
- Lymphadenopathy splenomegaly
- Local effects from tissue infiltration

Diagnosis
- Peripheral blood
- Bone marrow aspirate
- Flow cytometry
- Cytogenetics

Classify

Leukaemia = malignancy of bone marrow cells

Complicated classification
French American British (FAB) classification:
8 types of myeloid and 3 types of lymphoblastic

acute
- Acute lymphoblastic leukaemia (ALL)
- Acute myeloid leukaemia (AML)
- French American British (FAB classification) 8 types of myeloid and 3 types of lymphoblastic
- Immunological: (lymphoblastic) T-cell B-cell null-cell

chronic
- Chronic lymphatic leukaemia (CLL)
- Chronic myeloid leukaemia (CML)
- Hairy cell leukaemia

Complications
- Anaemia
- Haemorrhage
- Infections
- Metabolic abnormalities e.g. hypercalcaemia

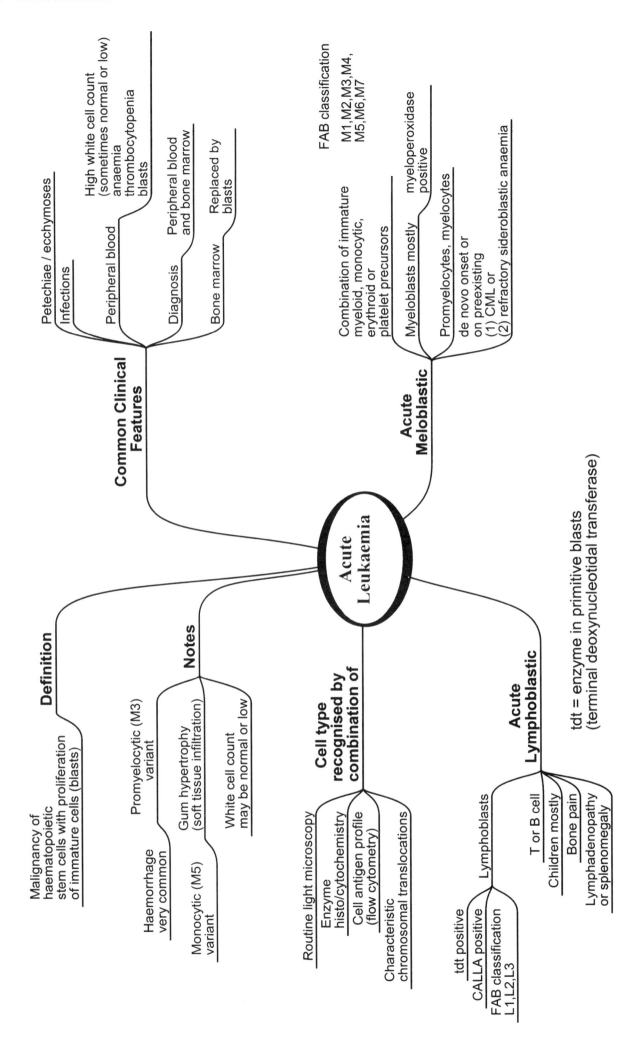

Acute Leukaemia

Common Clinical Features

Petechiae / ecchymoses

Infections

Peripheral blood — High white cell count (sometimes normal or low) anaemia thrombocytopenia blasts

Diagnosis — Peripheral blood and bone marrow

Bone marrow — Replaced by blasts

Acute Meloblastic

FAB classification M1,M2,M3,M4, M5,M6,M7

Combination of immature myeloid, monocytic, erythroid or platelet precursors

Myeloblasts mostly — myeloperoxidase positive

Promyelocytes, myelocytes

de novo onset or on preexisting
(1) CML or
(2) refractory sideroblastic anaemia

Definition

Malignancy of haematopoietic stem cells with proliferation of immature cells (blasts)

Notes

Haemorrhage very common

Promyelocytic (M3) variant

Monocytic (M5) variant — Gum hypertrophy (soft tissue infiltration)

White cell count may be normal or low

Cell type recognised by combination of

Routine light microscopy

Enzyme histo/cytochemistry

Cell antigen profile (flow cytometry)

Characteristic chromosomal translocations

Acute Lymphoblastic

Lymphoblasts — tdt positive, CALLA positive, FAB classification L1,L2,L3

T or B cell

Children mostly

Bone pain

Lymphadenopathy or splenomegaly

tdt = enzyme in primitive blasts (terminal deoxynucleotidal transferase)

Chronic Myeloid Leukaemia (CML)

Definition

Malignant proliferation of myeloid cells, showing varying degrees of maturation

Clinical

All ages
mostly adults

Massive splenomegaly (pain)

Gout

Indolent chronic phase followed by blast crisis (acute leukaemia)

Laboratory

Anaemia

Thrombocytosis followed by thrombocytopenia

Very high white cell count

High levels of neutrophils and their precursors, eosinophils, basophils

Philadelphia chromosome t(9;22) abl/bcr

Blast crisis

Marrow replaced by differentiating granulocytes (indistinguishable from granulocytic hyperplasia)

Chronic Leukaemia

CML

CLL

Chronic Lymphocytic Leukaemia (CLL)

Definition

Neoplastic proliferation of differentiated lymphocytes involving marrow and blood

Clinical

Lymphadenopathy splenomegaly

Middle age and elderly

Fatigue

Infections

Autoimmune haemolytic anaemia

Autoimmune thrombocytopenia

Staging

Depends on degrees of
lymphadenopathy
lymphocytosis
anaemia
thrombocytopenia

Binet system

Rai system

Laboratory

Lymphocytosis

B cells:
surface immunoglobulin
usually IgM or IgD,
CD5+, CD19+
CD20+, CD23+

Anaemia

Thrombocytopenia

Hypogammaglobulinaemia (25% pts)

Hypergammaglobulinaemia (10% pts)

Monoclonal gammopathy (5% pts)

Chromosomal abnormalities:
trisomy 12 (50% patients)
other abnormalities

Other Chronic (lymphoid) Leukaemias

Prolymphocytic
Hairy cell leukaemia
Sezary syndrome (leukaemic phase of Mycosis fungoides)
Waldenstrom's macroglobulinaemia

SYSTEMATIC PATHOLOGY

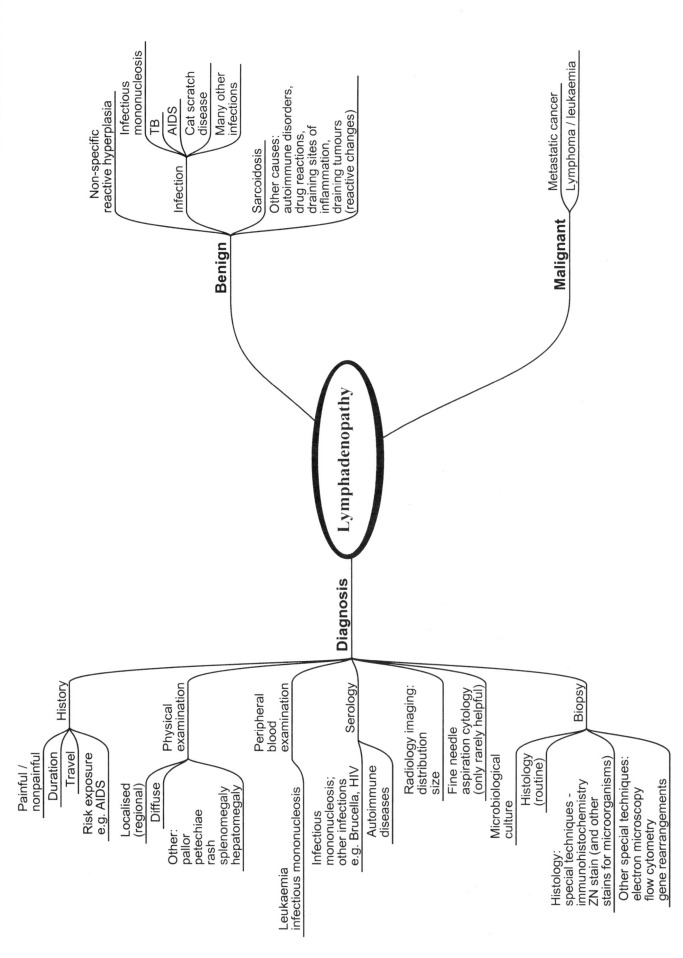

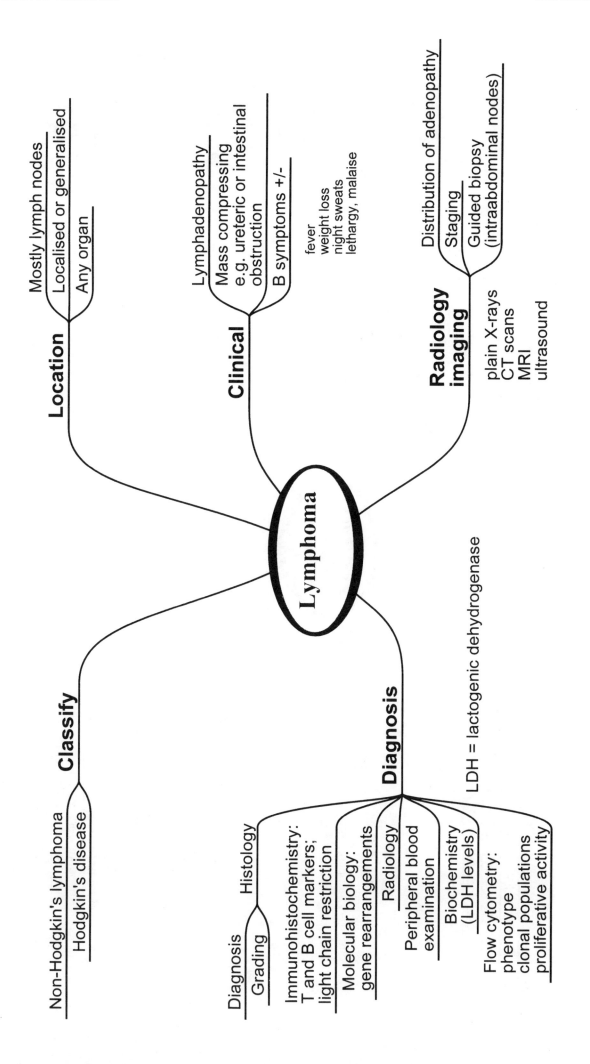

Lymphoma

Location
- Mostly lymph nodes
  - Localised or generalised
- Any organ

Clinical
- Lymphadenopathy
- Mass compressing e.g. ureteric or intestinal obstruction
- B symptoms +/-
  - fever
  - weight loss
  - night sweats
  - lethargy, malaise

Radiology imaging
- Distribution of adenopathy
  - Staging
  - Guided biopsy (intraabdominal nodes)
- plain X-rays
- CT scans
- MRI
- ultrasound

Classify
- Non-Hodgkin's lymphoma
- Hodgkin's disease

Diagnosis
- Histology
  - Diagnosis
  - Grading
- Immunohistochemistry: T and B cell markers; light chain restriction
- Molecular biology: gene rearrangements
- Radiology
- Peripheral blood examination
- Biochemistry (LDH levels)
- Flow cytometry: phenotype, clonal populations, proliferative activity
- LDH = lactogenic dehydrogenase

SYSTEMATIC PATHOLOGY

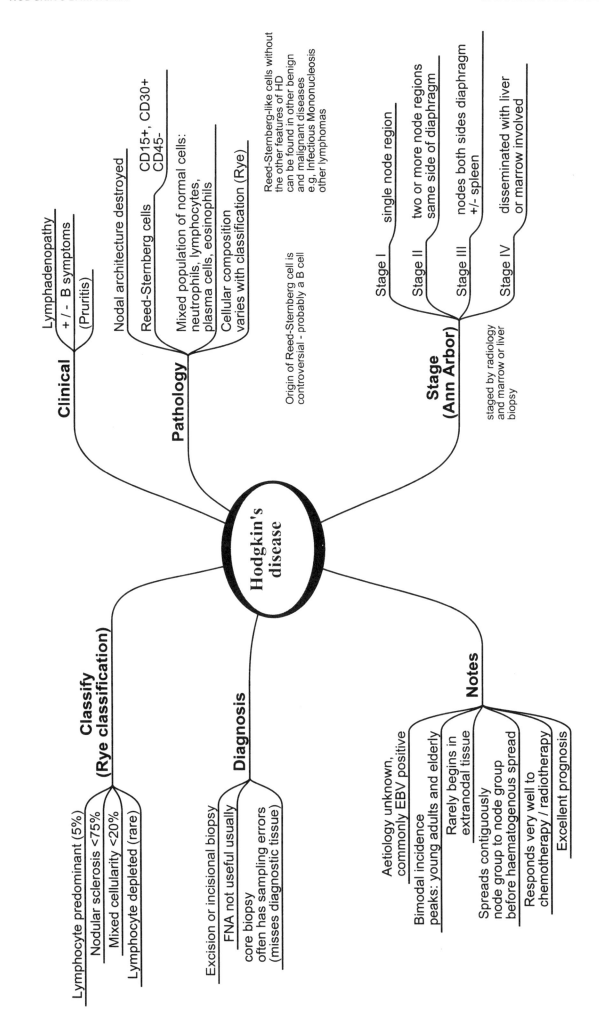

Hodgkin's disease

Clinical
- Lymphadenopathy
- +/− B symptoms
- (Pruritis)

Pathology
- Nodal architecture destroyed
- Reed-Sternberg cells — CD15+, CD30+ CD45−
- Mixed population of normal cells: neutrophils, lymphocytes, plasma cells, eosinophils
- Cellular composition varies with classification (Rye)

Origin of Reed-Sternberg cell is controversial - probably a B cell

Reed-Sternberg-like cells without the other features of HD can be found in other benign and malignant diseases e.g. Infectious Mononucleosis other lymphomas

Stage (Ann Arbor)
- Stage I — single node region
- Stage II — two or more node regions same side of diaphragm
- Stage III — nodes both sides diaphragm +/− spleen
- Stage IV — disseminated with liver or marrow involved

staged by radiology and marrow or liver biopsy

Classify (Rye classification)
- Lymphocyte predominant (5%)
- Nodular sclerosis <75%
- Mixed cellularity <20%
- Lymphocyte depleted (rare)

Diagnosis
- Excision or incisional biopsy
- FNA not useful usually core biopsy
- often has sampling errors (misses diagnostic tissue)

Notes
- Aetiology unknown, commonly EBV positive
- Bimodal incidence peaks: young adults and elderly
- Rarely begins in extranodal tissue
- Spreads contiguously node group to node group before haematogenous spread
- Responds very well to chemotherapy / radiotherapy
- Excellent prognosis

SYSTEMATIC PATHOLOGY

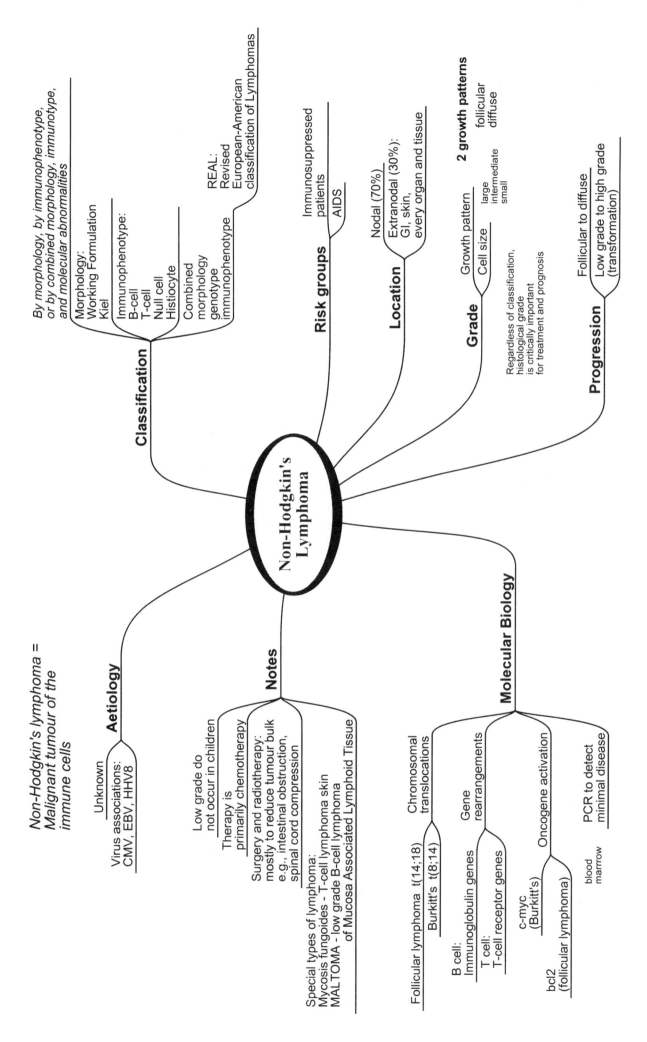

Non-Hodgkin's Lymphoma

Classification

By morphology, by immunophenotype, or by combined morphology, immunotype, and molecular abnormalities

Morphology:
Working Formulation
Kiel

Immunophenotype:
B-cell
T-cell
Null cell
Histiocyte

Combined morphology genotype immunophenotype

REAL: Revised European-American classification of Lymphomas

Risk groups

Immunosuppressed patients

AIDS

Location

Nodal (70%)

Extranodal (30%):
GI, skin, every organ and tissue

Grade

Growth pattern

Cell size
large
intermediate
small

Regardless of classification, histological grade is critically important for treatment and prognosis

2 growth patterns

follicular
diffuse

Progression

Follicular to diffuse

Low grade to high grade (transformation)

Non-Hodgkin's lymphoma = Malignant tumour of the immune cells

Aetiology

Unknown

Virus associations: CMV, EBV, HHV8

Notes

Low grade do not occur in children

Therapy is primarily chemotherapy

Surgery and radiotherapy: mostly to reduce tumour bulk e.g., intestinal obstruction, spinal cord compression

Special types of lymphoma:
Mycosis fungoides - T-cell lymphoma skin
MALTOMA - low grade B-cell lymphoma of Mucosa Associated Lymphoid Tissue

Molecular Biology

Chromosomal translocations

Follicular lymphoma t(14;18)

Burkitt's t(8;14)

Gene rearrangements

B cell:
Immunoglobulin genes

T cell:
T-cell receptor genes

Oncogene activation

c-myc (Burkitt's)

bcl2 (follicular lymphoma)

PCR to detect minimal disease

blood
marrrow

SYSTEMATIC PATHOLOGY

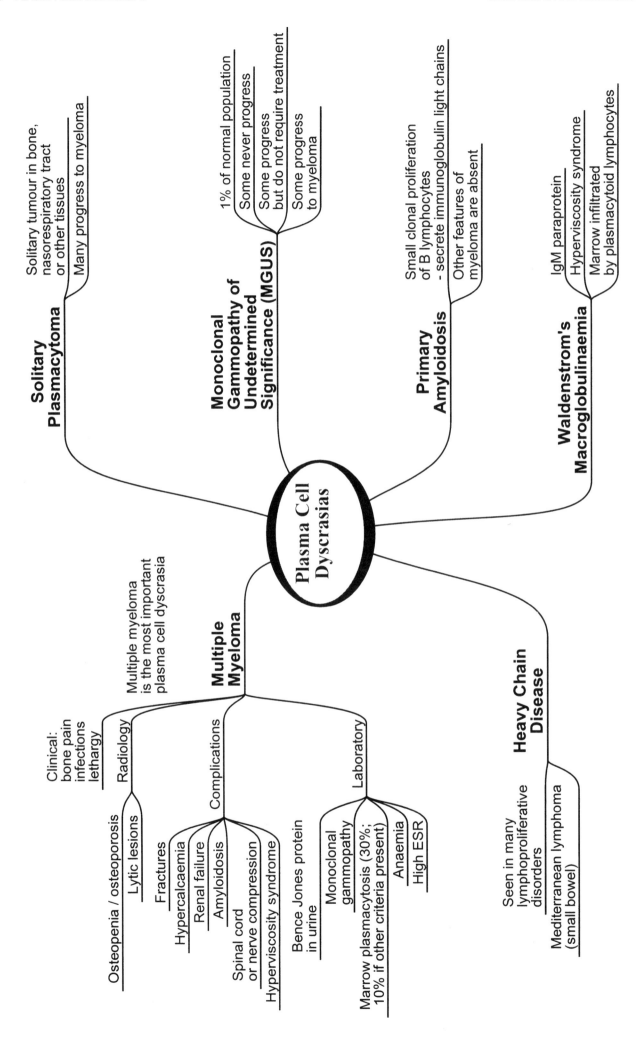

Plasma Cell Dyscrasias

Solitary Plasmacytoma
- Solitary tumour in bone, nasorespiratory tract or other tissues
- Many progress to myeloma

Monoclonal Gammopathy of Undetermined Significance (MGUS)
- 1% of normal population
- Some never progress
- Some progress but do not require treatment
- Some progress to myeloma

Primary Amyloidosis
- Small clonal proliferation of B lymphocytes - secrete immunoglobulin light chains
- Other features of myeloma are absent

Waldenstrom's Macroglobulinaemia
- IgM paraprotein
- Hyperviscosity syndrome
- Marrow infiltrated by plasmacytoid lymphocytes

Multiple Myeloma
- Multiple myeloma is the most important plasma cell dyscrasia
- Clinical: bone pain infections lethargy
- Radiology
  - Osteopenia / osteoporosis
  - Lytic lesions
  - Fractures
- Complications
  - Hypercalcaemia
  - Renal failure
  - Amyloidosis
  - Spinal cord or nerve compression
  - Hyperviscosity syndrome
- Laboratory
  - Bence Jones protein in urine
  - Monoclonal gammopathy
  - Marrow plasmacytosis (30%; 10% if other criteria present)
  - Anaemia
  - High ESR

Heavy Chain Disease
- Seen in many lymphoproliferative disorders
- Mediterranean lymphoma (small bowel)

BONES, JOINTS AND SOFT TISSUE TUMOURS

SYSTEMATIC PATHOLOGY

SYSTEMATIC PATHOLOGY

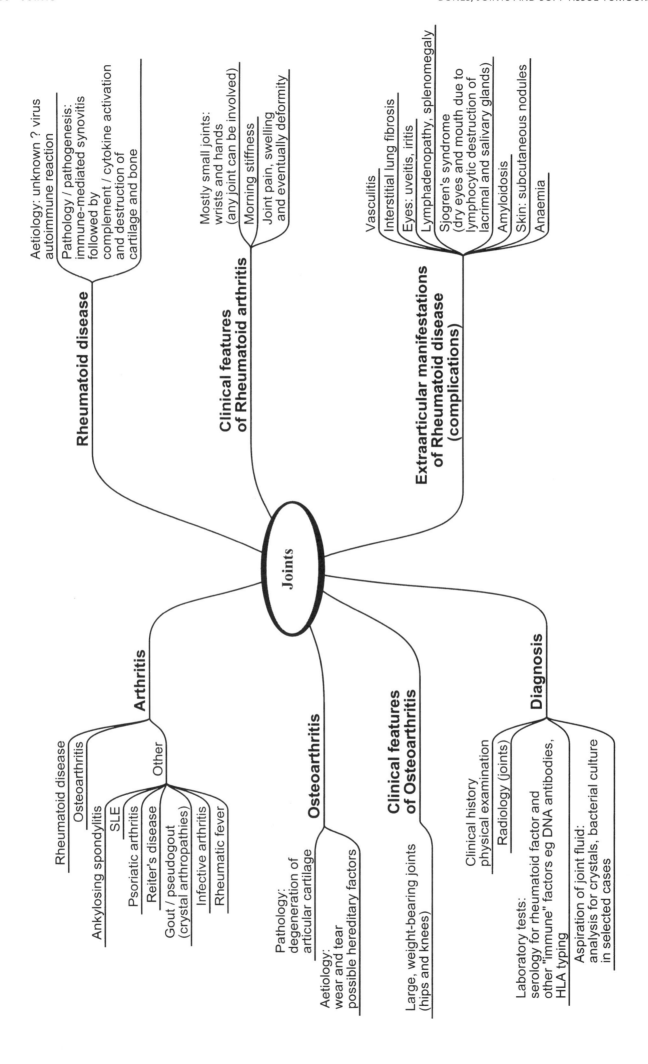

Joints

Rheumatoid disease

Aetiology: unknown ? virus autoimmune reaction

Pathology / pathogenesis: immune-mediated synovitis followed by complement / cytokine activation and destruction of cartilage and bone

Clinical features of Rheumatoid arthritis

Mostly small joints: wrists and hands (any joint can be involved)

Morning stiffness

Joint pain, swelling and eventually deformity

Extraarticular manifestations of Rheumatoid disease (complications)

Vasculitis

Interstitial lung fibrosis

Eyes: uveitis, iritis

Lymphadenopathy, splenomegaly

Sjogren's syndrome (dry eyes and mouth due to lymphocytic destruction of lacrimal and salivary glands)

Amyloidosis

Skin: subcutaneous nodules

Anaemia

Arthritis

Rheumatoid disease

Osteoarthritis

Ankylosing spondylitis

SLE

Psoriatic arthritis

Reiter's disease

Other

Gout / pseudogout (crystal arthropathies)

Infective arthritis

Rheumatic fever

Osteoarthritis

Pathology: degeneration of articular cartilage

Aetiology: wear and tear possible hereditary factors

Clinical features of Osteoarthritis

Large, weight-bearing joints (hips and knees)

Diagnosis

Clinical history physical examination

Radiology (joints)

Laboratory tests: serology for rheumatoid factor and other "immune" factors eg DNA antibodies, HLA typing

Aspiration of joint fluid: analysis for crystals, bacterial culture in selected cases

SYSTEMATIC PATHOLOGY

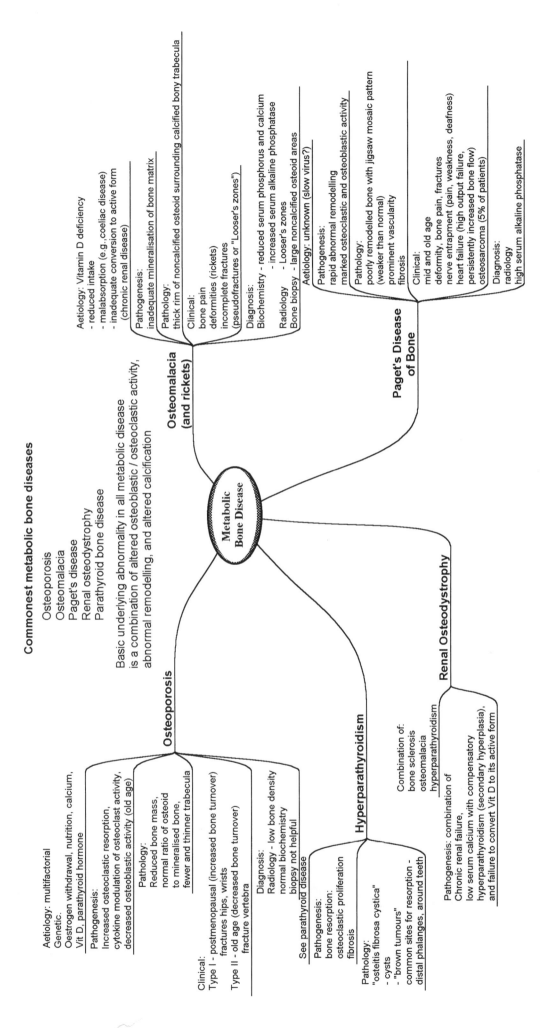

SYSTEMATIC PATHOLOGY

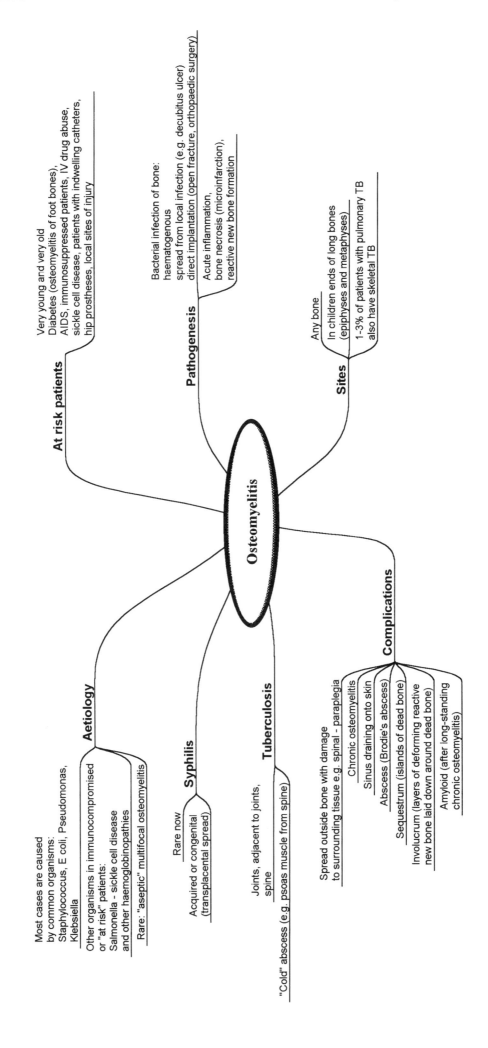

Osteomyelitis

At risk patients
- Very young and very old
- Diabetes (osteomyelitis of foot bones), AIDS, immunosuppressed patients, IV drug abuse, sickle cell disease, patients with indwelling catheters, hip prostheses, local sites of injury

Pathogenesis
- Bacterial infection of bone: haematogenous spread from local infection (e.g. decubitus ulcer) direct implantation (open fracture, orthopaedic surgery)
- Acute inflammation, bone necrosis (microinfarction), reactive new bone formation

Sites
- Any bone
- In children ends of long bones (epiphyses and metaphyses)
- 1-3% of patients with pulmonary TB also have skeletal TB

Aetiology
- Most cases are caused by common organisms: Staphylococcus, E coli, Pseudomonas, Klebsiella
- Other organisms in immunocompromised or "at risk" patients: Salmonella - sickle cell disease and other haemoglobinopathies
- Rare: "aseptic" multifocal osteomyelitis

Syphilis
- Rare now
- Acquired or congenital (transplacental spread)

Tuberculosis
- Joints, adjacent to joints, spine
- "Cold" abscess (e.g. psoas muscle from spine)

Complications
- Spread outside bone with damage to surrounding tissue e.g. spinal - paraplegia
- Chronic osteomyelitis
- Sinus draining onto skin
- Abscess (Brodie's abscess)
- Sequestrum (islands of dead bone)
- Involucrum (layers of deforming reactive new bone laid down around dead bone)
- Amyloid (after long-standing chronic osteomyelitis)

SYSTEMATIC PATHOLOGY

Bone Tumours

Primary tumours

Benign
- Osteoma
  osteoid osteoma
  osteoblastoma
- Osteochondroma
  enchondroma
- Giant cell tumour
- Other

Malignant
- Osteosarcoma
- Chondrosarcoma
- Ewing's sarcoma
- Other:
  fibrosarcoma
  lymphoma
  malignant fibrous histiocytoma
- Malignant giant cell tumour
- Local invasion
  – bone and soft tissue
- Haematogenous metastases
  – typically lung

Malignancy in pre-existing disease
- Paget's Disease
- Hereditary Retinoblastoma
- Multiple Chondromas
- Giant Cell Tumour

Metastatic
- Lung
- Prostate
- Breast
- Others

Metastatic cancers to bone are much commoner than primary bone cancers

Diagnosis

Radiology
- Plain X-ray
- CT
- MRI

Evaluates location, size, pattern of bone destruction or reaction

Biopsy

Clinical
- Pain

Age Groups:
children:
osteosarcoma, Ewing's sarcoma;
adults:
chondrosarcoma

Tumour-like lesions:
cysts: may look like tumour on X-ray, in particular, osteomyelitis may resemble Ewing's

SYSTEMATIC PATHOLOGY

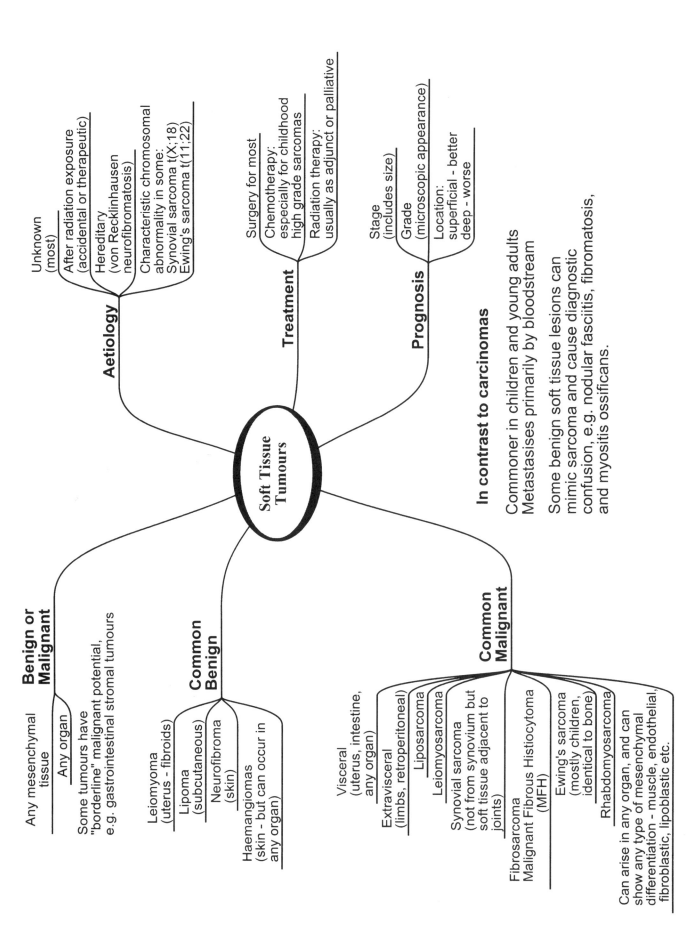

Aetiology

Unknown (most)

After radiation exposure (accidental or therapeutic)

Hereditary (von Recklinghausen neurofibromatosis)

Characteristic chromosomal abnormality in some:
Synovial sarcoma t(X;18)
Ewing's sarcoma t(11;22)

Treatment

Surgery for most

Chemotherapy: especially for childhood high grade sarcomas

Radiation therapy: usually as adjunct or palliative

Prognosis

Stage (includes size)

Grade (microscopic appearance)

Location: superficial - better deep - worse

Soft Tissue Tumours

In contrast to carcinomas

Commoner in children and young adults
Metastasises primarily by bloodstream

Some benign soft tissue lesions can mimic sarcoma and cause diagnostic confusion, e.g. nodular fasciitis, fibromatosis, and myositis ossificans.

Benign or Malignant

Any mesenchymal tissue

Any organ

Some tumours have "borderline" malignant potential, e.g. gastrointestinal stromal tumours

Common Benign

Leiomyoma (uterus - fibroids)

Lipoma (subcutaneous)

Neurofibroma (skin)

Haemangiomas (skin - but can occur in any organ)

Common Malignant

Visceral (uterus, intestine, any organ)

Extravisceral (limbs, retroperitoneal)

Liposarcoma

Leiomyosarcoma

Synovial sarcoma (not from synovium but soft tissue adjacent to joints)

Fibrosarcoma

Malignant Fibrous Histiocytoma (MFH)

Ewing's sarcoma (mostly children, identical to bone)

Rhabdomyosarcoma

Can arise in any organ, and can show any type of mesenchymal differentiation - muscle, endothelial, fibroblastic, lipoblastic etc.

SKIN

SYSTEMATIC PATHOLOGY

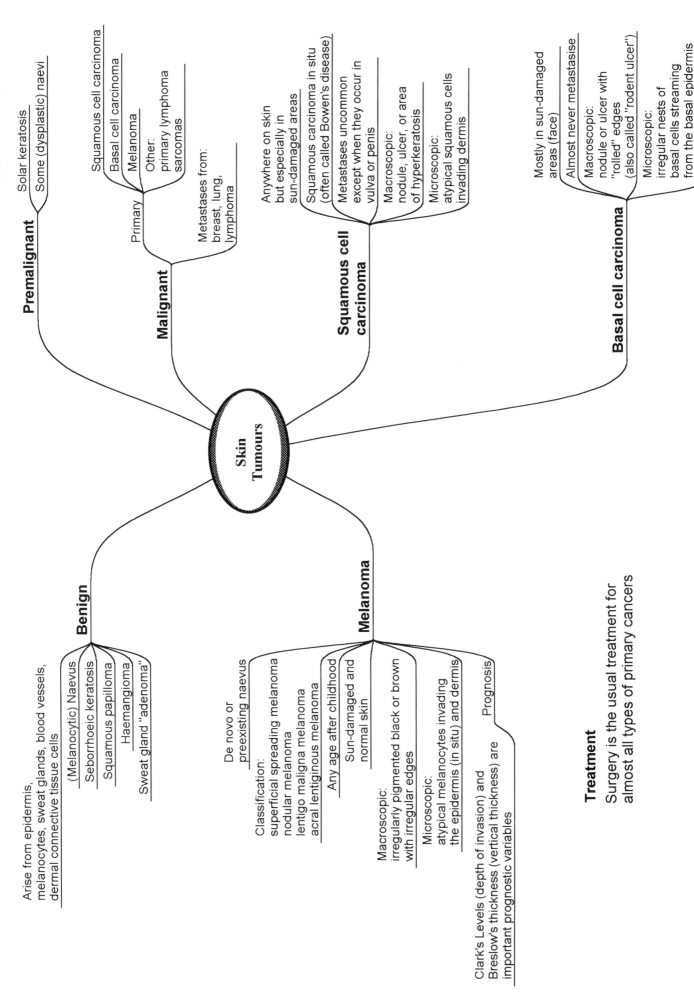

Skin Tumours

Premalignant
- Solar keratosis
- Some (dysplastic) naevi

Malignant
- Primary
  - Squamous cell carcinoma
  - Basal cell carcinoma
  - Melanoma
  - Other: primary lymphoma sarcomas
- Metastases from: breast, lung, lymphoma

Squamous cell carcinoma
- Anywhere on skin but especially in sun-damaged areas
- Squamous carcinoma in situ (often called Bowen's disease)
- Metastases uncommon except when they occur in vulva or penis
- Macroscopic: nodule, ulcer, or area of hyperkeratosis
- Microscopic: atypical squamous cells invading dermis

Basal cell carcinoma
- Mostly in sun-damaged areas (face)
- Almost never metastasise
- Macroscopic: nodule or ulcer with "rolled" edges (also called "rodent ulcer")
- Microscopic: irregular nests of basal cells streaming from the basal epidermis into the dermis (invasion)

Benign
- Arise from epidermis, melanocytes, sweat glands, blood vessels, dermal connective tissue cells
  - (Melanocytic) Naevus
  - Seborrhoeic keratosis
  - Squamous papilloma
  - Haemangioma
  - Sweat gland "adenoma"

Melanoma
- De novo or preexisting naevus
- Classification: superficial spreading melanoma nodular melanoma lentigo maligna melanoma acral lentiginous melanoma
- Any age after childhood
- Sun-damaged and normal skin
- Macroscopic: irregularly pigmented black or brown with irregular edges
- Microscopic: atypical melanocytes invading the epidermis (in situ) and dermis
- Prognosis
  - Clark's Levels (depth of invasion) and Breslow's thickness (vertical thickness) are important prognostic variables

Treatment
Surgery is the usual treatment for almost all types of primary cancers

HEAD AND NECK

SYSTEMATIC PATHOLOGY

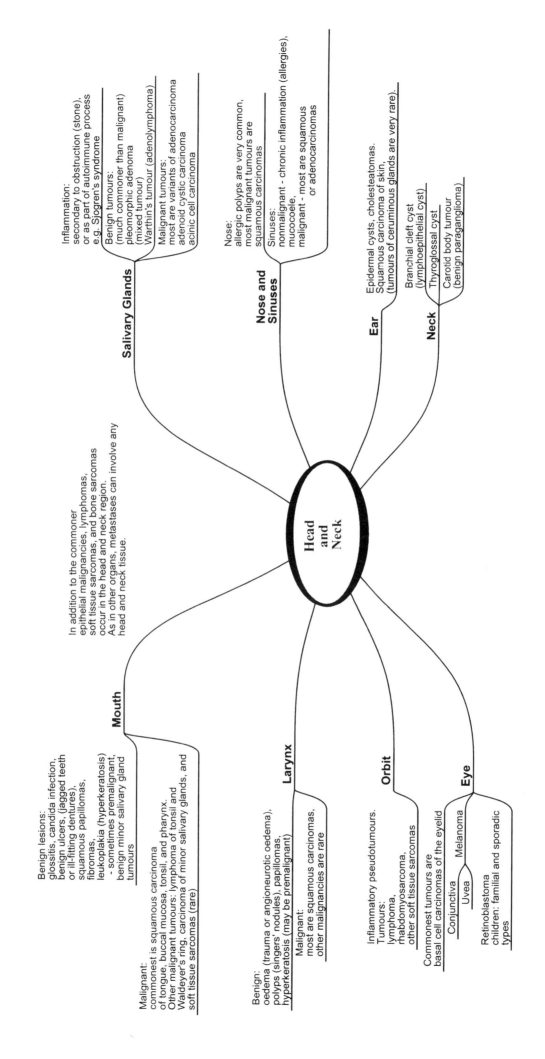

Salivary Glands

Inflammation:
secondary to obstruction (stone),
or as part of autoimmune process
e.g. Sjögren's syndrome

Benign tumours:
(much commoner than malignant)
pleomorphic adenoma
(mixed tumour)
Warthin's tumour (adenolymphoma)

Malignant tumours:
most are variants of adenocarcinoma
adenoid cystic carcinoma
acinic cell carcinoma

Nose and Sinuses

Nose:
allergic polyps are very common,
most malignant tumours are
squamous carcinomas

Sinuses:
nonmalignant - chronic inflammation (allergies),
mucocoele,
malignant - most are squamous
or adenocarcinomas

Ear

Epidermal cysts, cholesteatomas.
Squamous carcinoma of skin,
(tumours of ceruminous glands are very rare).

Neck

Branchial cleft cyst
(lymphoepithelial cyst)
Thyroglossal cyst
Carotid body tumour
(benign paraganglioma)

Head and Neck

In addition to the commoner
epithelial malignancies, lymphomas,
soft tissue sarcomas, and bone sarcomas
occur in the head and neck region.
As in other organs, metastases can involve any
head and neck tissue.

Mouth

Benign lesions:
glossitis, candida infection,
benign ulcers, (jagged teeth
or ill-fitting dentures),
squamous papillomas,
fibromas,
leukoplakia (hyperkeratosis)
- sometimes premalignant,
benign minor salivary gland
tumours

Malignant:
commonest is squamous carcinoma
of tongue, buccal mucosa, tonsil, and pharynx.
Other malignant tumours: lymphoma of tonsil and
Waldeyer's ring, carcinoma of minor salivary glands, and
soft tissue sarcomas (rare)

Larynx

Benign:
oedema (trauma or angioneurotic oedema),
polyps (singers' nodules), papillomas,
hyperkeratosis (may be premalignant)

Malignant:
most are squamous carcinomas,
other malignancies are rare

Orbit

Inflammatory pseudotumours.
Tumours:
lymphoma,
rhabdomyosarcoma,
other soft tissue sarcomas

Eye

Commonest tumours are
basal cell carcinomas of the eyelid

Conjunctiva   Melanoma
        Uvea

Retinoblastoma
children: familial and sporadic
types

CENTRAL AND PERIPHERAL NERVOUS SYSTEM

SYSTEMATIC PATHOLOGY

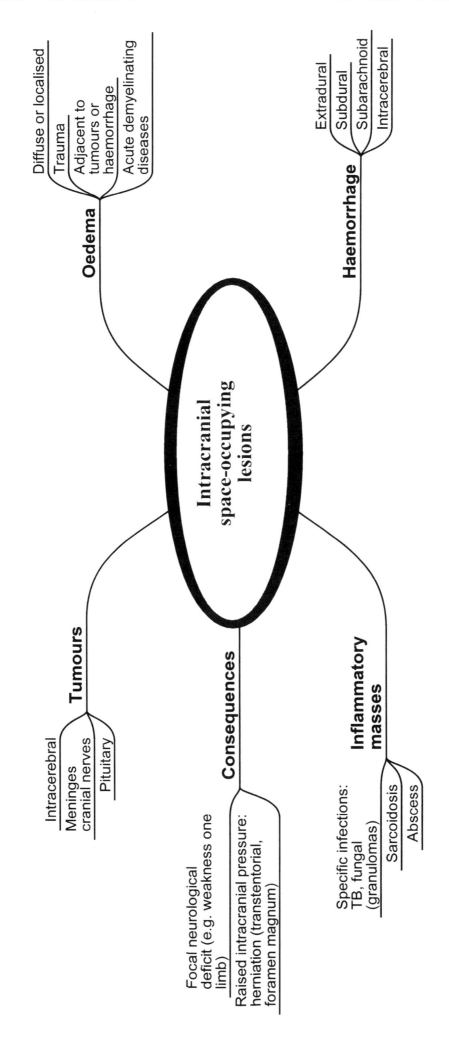

Intracranial space-occupying lesions

Oedema
- Diffuse or localised
- Trauma
- Adjacent to tumours or haemorrhage
- Acute demyelinating diseases

Haemorrhage
- Extradural
- Subdural
- Subarachnoid
- Intracerebral

Tumours
- Intracerebral
- Meninges
- cranial nerves
- Pituitary

Consequences
- Focal neurological deficit (e.g. weakness one limb)
- Raised intracranial pressure: herniation (transtentorial, foramen magnum)

Inflammatory masses
- Specific infections: TB, fungal (granulomas)
- Sarcoidosis
- Abscess

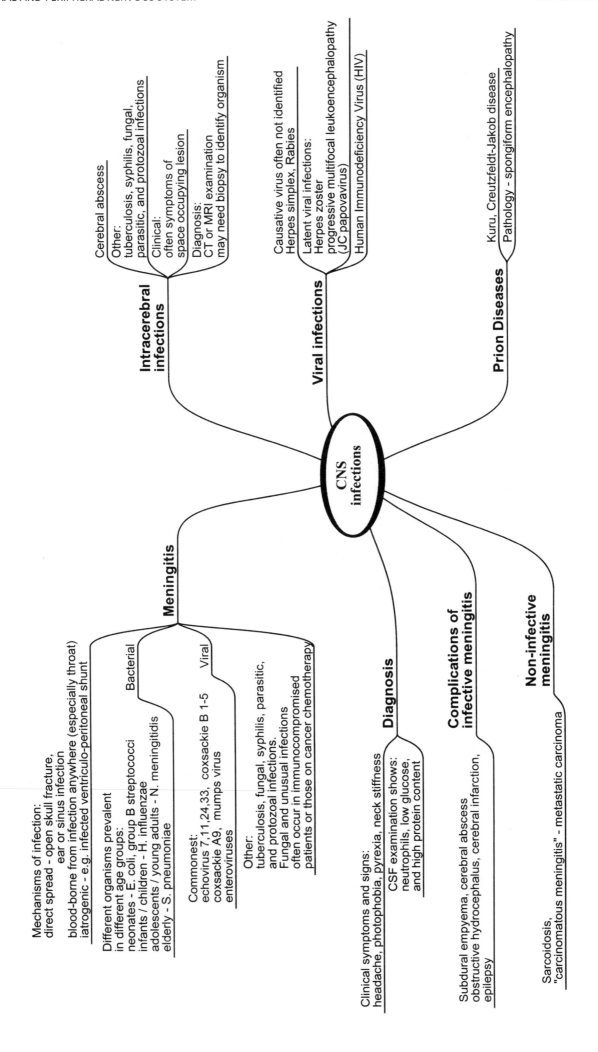

CNS infections

Intracerebral infections

Cerebral abscess

Other:
tuberculosis, syphilis, fungal, parasitic, and protozoal infections

Clinical:
often symptoms of space occupying lesion

Diagnosis:
CT or MRI examination
may need biopsy to identify organism

Viral infections

Causative virus often not identified
Herpes simplex, Rabies

Latent viral infections:
Herpes zoster
progressive multifocal leukoencephalopathy (JC papovavirus)

Human Immunodeficiency Virus (HIV)

Prion Diseases

Kuru, Creutzfeldt-Jakob disease

Pathology - spongiform encephalopathy

Meningitis

Mechanisms of infection:
direct spread - open skull fracture,
ear or sinus infection
blood-borne from infection anywhere (especially throat)
iatrogenic - e.g. infected ventriculo-peritoneal shunt

Different organisms prevalent
in different age groups:
neonates - E. coli, group B streptococci
infants / children - H. influenzae
adolescents / young adults - N. meningitidis
elderly - S. pneumoniae

Bacterial

Commonest:
echovirus 7,11,24,33, coxsackie B 1-5
coxsackie A9, mumps virus
enteroviruses

Viral

Other:
tuberculosis, fungal, syphilis, parasitic,
and protozoal infections.
Fungal and unusual infections
often occur in immunocompromised
patients or those on cancer chemotherapy

Diagnosis

Clinical symptoms and signs:
headache, photophobia, pyrexia, neck stiffness

CSF examination shows:
neutrophils, low glucose,
and high protein content

Complications of infective meningitis

Subdural empyema, cerebral abscess
obstructive hydrocephalus, cerebral infarction,
epilepsy

Non-infective meningitis

Sarcoidosis,
"carcinomatous meningitis" - metastatic carcinoma

SYSTEMATIC PATHOLOGY

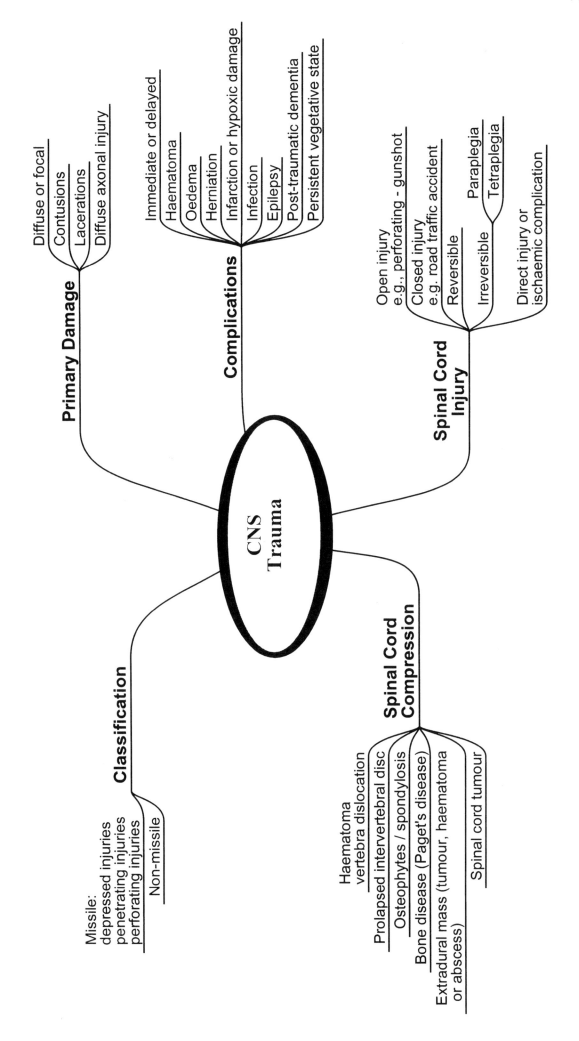

Primary Damage
- Diffuse or focal
- Contusions
- Lacerations
- Diffuse axonal injury

Complications
- Immediate or delayed
- Haematoma
- Oedema
- Herniation
- Infarction or hypoxic damage
- Infection
- Epilepsy
- Post-traumatic dementia
- Persistent vegetative state

Spinal Cord Injury
- Open injury e.g., perforating - gunshot
- Closed injury e.g. road traffic accident
- Reversible
- Irreversible
  - Paraplegia
  - Tetraplegia
- Direct injury or ischaemic complication

Classification
- Missile: depressed injuries, penetrating injuries, perforating injuries
- Non-missile

Spinal Cord Compression
- Haematoma
- vertebra dislocation
- Prolapsed intervertebral disc
- Osteophytes / spondylosis
- Bone disease (Paget's disease)
- Extradural mass (tumour, haematoma or abscess)
- Spinal cord tumour

CNS Trauma

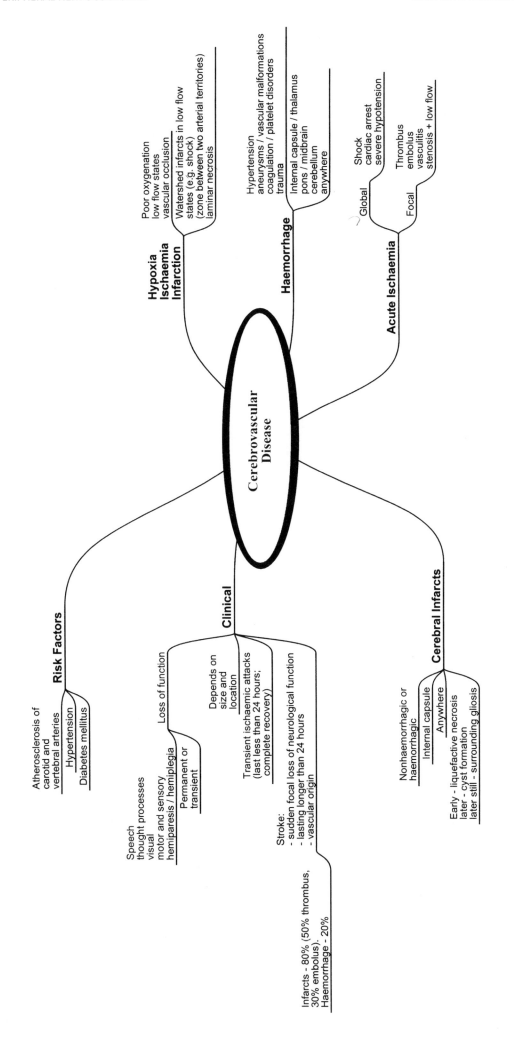

Cerebrovascular Disease

Hypoxia Ischaemia Infarction
- Poor oxygenation
- low flow states
- vascular occlusion
- Watershed infarcts in low flow states (e.g. shock) (zone between two arterial territories)
- laminar necrosis

Haemorrhage
- Hypertension
- aneurysms / vascular malformations
- coagulation / platelet disorders
- trauma
- Internal capsule / thalamus
- pons / midbrain
- cerebellum
- anywhere

Acute Ischaemia
- Global
  - Shock
  - cardiac arrest
  - severe hypotension
- Focal
  - Thrombus
  - embolus
  - vasculitis
  - stenosis + low flow

Risk Factors
- Atherosclerosis of carotid and vertebral arteries
- Hypertension
- Diabetes mellitus

Clinical
- Loss of function
  - Speech
  - thought processes
  - visual
  - motor and sensory
  - hemiparesis / hemiplegia
  - Permanent or transient
- Depends on size and location
- Transient ischaemic attacks (last less than 24 hours; complete recovery)
- Stroke:
  - sudden focal loss of neurological function
  - lasting longer than 24 hours
  - vascular origin
- Infarcts - 80% (50% thrombus, 30% embolus).
- Haemorrhage - 20%

Cerebral Infarcts
- Nonhaemorrhagic or haemorrhagic
- Internal capsule
- Anywhere
- Early - liquefactive necrosis
- later - cyst formation
- later still - surrounding gliosis

SYSTEMATIC PATHOLOGY

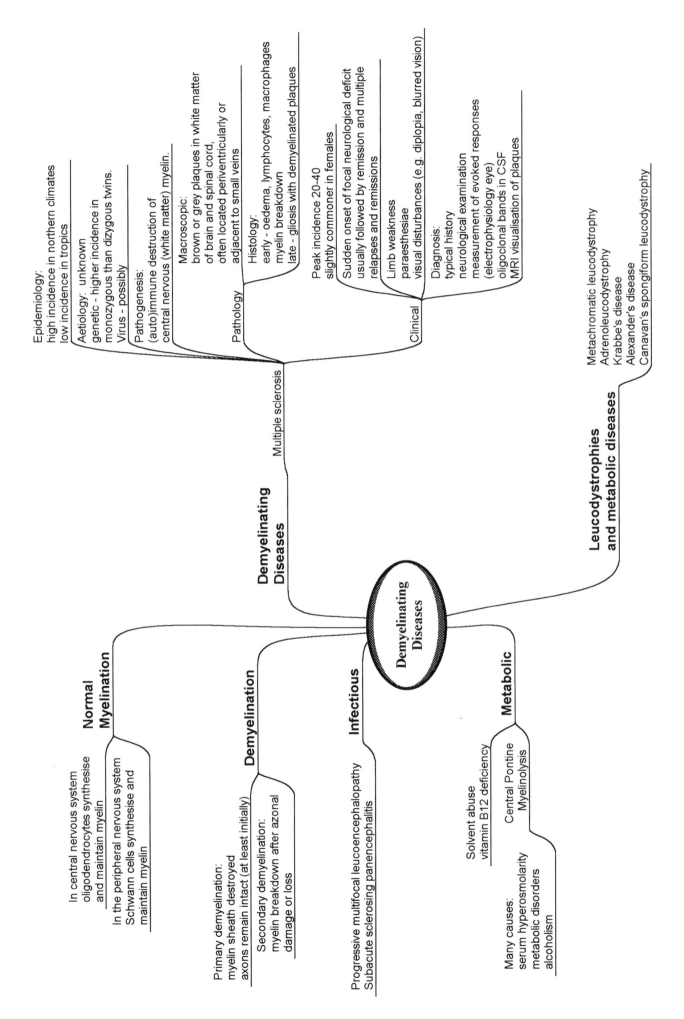

Demyelinating Diseases

Demyelinating Diseases

Multiple sclerosis

Epidemiology:
high incidence in northern climates
low incidence in tropics

Aetiology: unknown
genetic - higher incidence in
monozygous than dizygous twins.
Virus - possibly

Pathogenesis:
(auto)immune destruction of
central nervous (white matter) myelin.

Pathology

Macroscopic:
brown or grey plaques in white matter
of brain and spinal cord,
often located periventricularly or
adjacent to small veins

Histology:
early - oedema, lymphocytes, macrophages
myelin breakdown
late - gliosis with demyelinated plaques

Clinical

Peak incidence 20-40
slightly commoner in females

Sudden onset of focal neurological deficit
usually followed by remission and multiple
relapses and remissions

Limb weakness
paraesthesie
visual disturbances (e.g. diplopia, blurred vision)

Diagnosis:
typical history
neurological examination
measurement of evoked responses
(electrophysiology eye)
oligoclonal bands in CSF
MRI visualisation of plaques

Leucodystrophies and metabolic diseases

Metachromatic leucodystrophy
Adrenoleucodystrophy
Krabbe's disease
Alexander's disease
Canavan's spongiform leucodystrophy

Normal Myelination

In central nervous system
oligodendrocytes synthesise
and maintain myelin

In the peripheral nervous system
Schwann cells synthesise and
maintain myelin

Demyelination

Primary demyelination:
myelin sheath destroyed
axons remain intact (at least initially)

Secondary demyelination:
myelin breakdown after azonal
damage or loss

Infectious

Progressive multifocal leucoencephalopathy
Subacute sclerosing panencephalitis

Metabolic

Solvent abuse
vitamin B12 deficiency

Central Pontine
Myelinolysis

Many causes:
serum hyperosmolarity
metabolic disorders
alcoholism

SYSTEMATIC PATHOLOGY

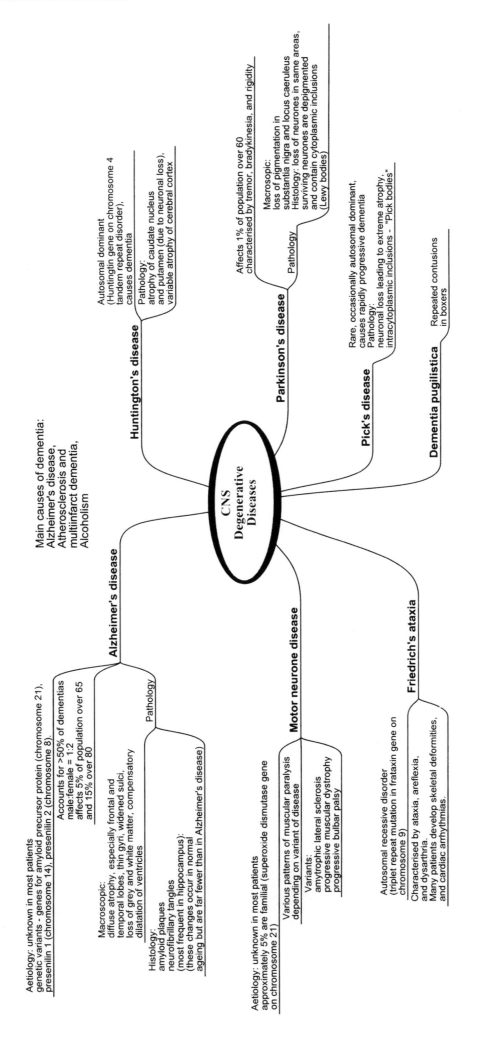

CNS Degenerative Diseases

Alzheimer's disease

Aetiology: unknown in most patients
genetic variants - genes for amyloid precursor protein (chromosome 21),
presenilin 1 (chromosome 14), presenilin 2 (chromosome 8).

Accounts for >50% of dementias
male:female = 1:2
affects 5% of population over 65
and 15% over 80

Main causes of dementia:
Alzheimer's disease,
Atherosclerosis and
multiinfarct dementia,
Alcoholism

Pathology

Macroscopic:
diffuse atrophy, especially frontal and
temporal lobes, thin gyri, widened sulci,
loss of grey and white matter, compensatory
dilatation of ventricles

Histology:
amyloid plaques
neurofibrillary tangles
(most frequent in hippocampus):
(these changes occur in normal
ageing but are far fewer than in Alzheimer's disease)

Huntington's disease

Autosomal dominant
(Huntingtin gene on chromosome 4
tandem repeat disorder),
causes dementia

Pathology:
atrophy of caudate nucleus
and putamen (due to neuronal loss),
variable atrophy of cerebral cortex

Parkinson's disease

Affects 1% of population over 60
characterised by tremor, bradykinesia, and rigidity

Pathology

Macroscopic:
loss of pigmentation in
substantia nigra and locus caeruleus
Histology: loss of neurones in same areas,
surviving neurones are depigmented
and contain cytoplasmic inclusions
(Lewy bodies)

Pick's disease

Rare, occasionally autosomal dominant,
causes rapidly progressive dementia
Pathology:
neuronal loss leading to extreme atrophy,
intracytoplasmic inclusions – "Pick bodies"

Dementia pugilistica

Repeated contusions
in boxers

Motor neurone disease

Aetiology: unknown in most patients
approximately 5% are familial (superoxide dismutase gene
on chromosome 21)

Various patterns of muscular paralysis
depending on variant of disease

Variants:
amytrophic lateral sclerosis
progressive muscular dystrophy
progressive bulbar palsy

Friedrich's ataxia

Autosomal recessive disorder
(triplet repeat mutation in frataxin gene on
chromosome 9)

Characterised by ataxia, areflexia,
and dysarthria.
Many patients develop skeletal deformities,
and cardiac arrhythmias.

SYSTEMATIC PATHOLOGY

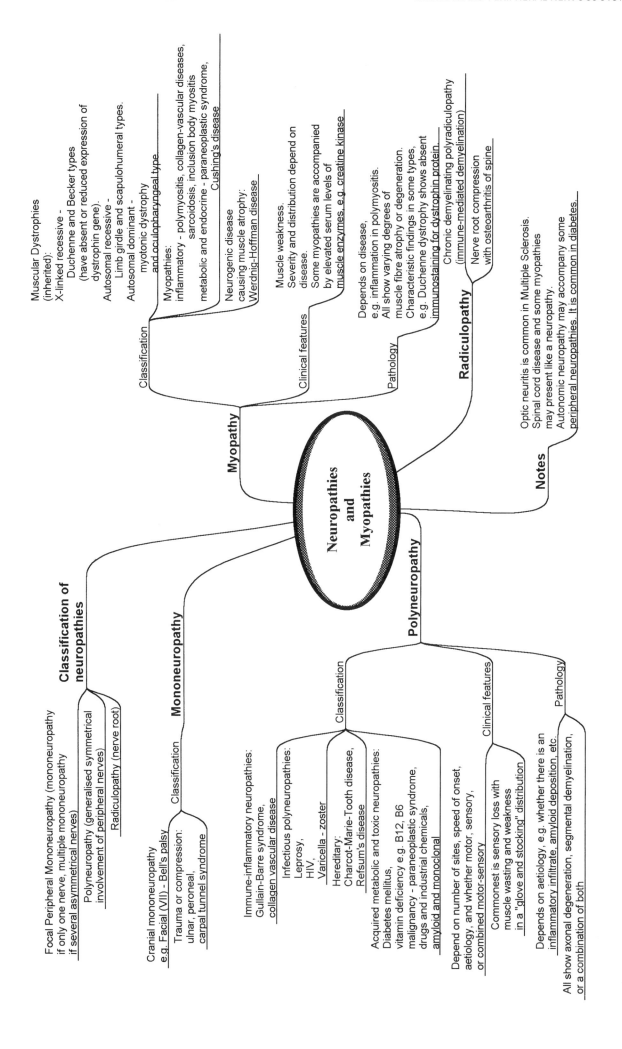

Myopathy

Classification

Muscular Dystrophies
(inherited):
- X-linked recessive -
  Duchenne and Becker types
  (have absent or reduced expression of
  dystrophin gene).
- Autosomal recessive -
  Limb girdle and scapulohumeral types.
- Autosomal dominant -
  myotonic dystrophy
  and oculopharyngeal type.

Myopathies:
inflammatory - polymyositis, collagen-vascular diseases,
sarcoidosis, inclusion body myositis
metabolic and endocrine - paraneoplastic syndrome,
Cushing's disease

Neurogenic disease
causing muscle atrophy:
Werdnig-Hoffman disease

Clinical features

Muscle weakness.
Severity and distribution depend on
disease.
Some myopathies are accompanied
by elevated serum levels of
muscle enzymes, e.g. creatine kinase

Pathology

Depends on disease,
e.g. inflammation in polymyositis.
All show varying degrees of
muscle fibre atrophy or degeneration.
Characteristic findings in some types,
e.g. Duchenne dystrophy shows absent
immunostaining for dystrophin protein.

Radiculopathy

Chronic demyelinating polyradiculopathy
(immune-mediated demyelination)

Nerve root compression
with osteoarthritis of spine

Notes

Optic neuritis is common in Multiple Sclerosis.
Spinal cord disease and some myopathies
may present like a neuropathy.
Autonomic neuropathy may accompany some
peripheral neuropathies. It is common in diabetes.

Classification of neuropathies

Classification

Focal Peripheral Mononeuropathy (mononeuropathy
if only one nerve, multiple mononeuropathy
if several asymmetrical nerves)

Polyneuropathy (generalised symmetrical
involvement of peripheral nerves)

Radiculopathy (nerve root)

Mononeuropathy

Classification

Cranial mononeuropathy
e.g. Facial (VII) - Bell's palsy

Trauma or compression:
ulnar, peroneal,
carpal tunnel syndrome

Neuropathies and Myopathies

Polyneuropathy

Classification

Immune-inflammatory neuropathies:
Gullain-Barre syndrome,
collagen vascular disease

Infectious polyneuropathies:
Leprosy,
HIV,
Varicella – zoster

Hereditary:
Charcot-Marie-Tooth disease,
Refsum's disease

Acquired metabolic and toxic neuropathies:
Diabetes mellitus,
vitamin deficiency e.g. B12, B6
malignancy - paraneoplastic syndrome,
drugs and industrial chemicals,
amyloid and monoclonal

Clinical features

Depend on number of sites, speed of onset,
aetiology, and whether motor, sensory,
or combined motor-sensory

Commonest is sensory loss with
muscle wasting and weakness
in a "glove and stocking" distribution

Pathology

Depends on aetiology, e.g. whether there is an
inflammatory infiltrate, amyloid deposition, etc.

All show axonal degeneration, segmental demyelination,
or a combination of both

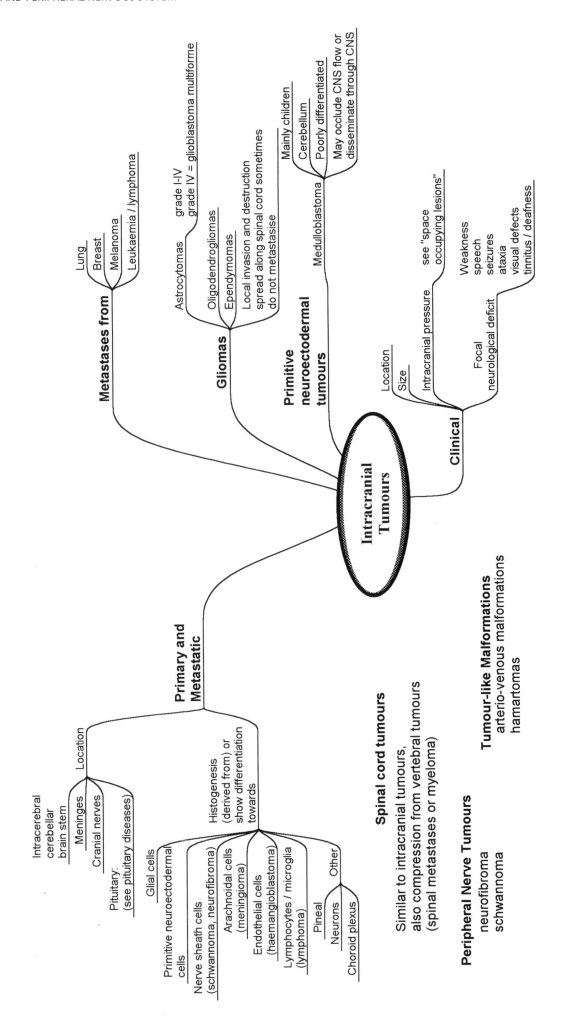

Intracranial Tumours

Metastases from
- Lung
- Breast
- Melanoma
- Leukaemia / lymphoma

Gliomas
- Astrocytomas — grade I-IV — grade IV = glioblastoma multiforme
- Oligodendrogliomas
- Ependymomas
- Local invasion and destruction spread along spinal cord sometimes do not metastasise

Primitive neuroectodermal tumours
- Medulloblastoma
  - Mainly children
  - Cerebellum
  - Poorly differentiated
  - May occlude CNS flow or disseminate through CNS

Clinical
- Location
- Size
- Intracranial pressure — see "space occupying lesions"
- Focal neurological deficit
  - Weakness
  - speech
  - seizures
  - ataxia
  - visual defects
  - tinnitus / deafness

Primary and Metastatic
- Location
  - Intracerebral
  - cerebellar
  - brain stem
  - Meninges
  - Cranial nerves
  - Pituitary: (see pituitary diseases)
- Histogenesis (derived from) or show differentiation towards
  - Glial cells
  - Primitive neuroectodermal cells
  - Nerve sheath cells (schwannoma, neurofibroma)
  - Arachnoidal cells (meningioma)
  - Endothelial cells (haemangioblastoma)
  - Lymphocytes / microglia (lymphoma)
  - Pineal
  - Neurons
  - Choroid plexus
  - Other

Spinal cord tumours
Similar to intracranial tumours, also compression from vertebral tumours (spinal metastases or myeloma)

Peripheral Nerve Tumours
neurofibroma
schwannoma

Tumour-like Malformations
arterio-venous malformations
hamartomas